NOURISH

The sustainable way to a healthier you

DOMINIC MUNNELLY has a degree in sports science backed up by 20 years of working in the health and fitness industry. He is a highly respected trainer, known for his knowledgeable, direct, no-bull but compassionate approach to getting you fit and healthy. He has appeared on television and spoken on radio frequently and has worked with hundreds of clients of all ages, shapes and fitness abilities.

Keep up to date with Dominic at:

🌐 www.thisitheway.ie
f Dominic Munnelly Personal Training
🐦 @dominicmunnelly
📷 dominicmunnelly

GRÁINNE PARKER is a graduate of Trinity College Dublin, has spent most of her working life in business consulting and has a deep understanding of the challenges of combining a busy working life and fitting in time for fitness and recreation activities. She has completed the professional three-month cookery course at Dublin Cookery School and has qualified as a health and wellness coach with the Institute of Health Sciences.

Keep up to date with Gráinne at:

🐦 @oliveoillemon (named for her two favourite ingredients)
📷 grainnehealthcoach

This book is for Eva who has lit up our lives since she arrived.

Thanks:

To our friends and family who encourage and support us every day in all that we do. Thank you to Mark, Ben and Edel, who were so very generous to us in lending us their lovely homes for photographs. To So&So, a wonderful Irish company who worked with us to develop our brand and book design. We could not recommend them more – highly creative, clever and so good at what they do.

Thanks to Cliodhna, our workout partner and lovely assistant.

To Larry of Laurence J Photography who took the photographs of us. Thank you for your lovely work and support.

To The Performance and Fitness Academy for use of the gym for photographs.

Finally, thank you to everyone over the years who has told us how much you like our recipes or how much Dominic has helped them get fit and become healthier.

MOVE
TRAIN
NOURISH

The sustainable way
to a healthier you

Dominic Munnelly & Gráinne Parker

The Collins Press

Disclaimer

Any health-related food or exercise advice is not intended as personal advice that you should follow without prior approval from your medical professional.

Consult a doctor before doing any of the exercises in this book.

It is your responsibility to evaluate your own medical and physical condition, and to independently determine whether to perform, use or adapt any of the information in this book. Any exercise programme may result in injury.

By voluntarily undertaking any exercise displayed in this book, you assume the risk of any resulting injury.

First published in 2018 by
The Collins Press
West Link Park
Doughcloyne
Wilton
Cork
T12 N5EF
Ireland

Photographs © Dominic Munnelly & Gráinne Parker except for pp 24, 31, 42 92, 93 and 108 which are © Shutterstock.

Dominic Munnelly & Gráinne Parker have asserted their moral right to be identified as the authors of this work in accordance with the Irish Copyright and Related Rights Act 2000.

A CIP record for this book is available from the British Library.

Paperback ISBN: 978-1-84889-335-1

Food styling and photography by Gráinne Parker

Exercise illustrations by Derry Dillon

Design and print origination by Fairways Design
Based on an original design by So&So
Typeset in Flama and Lexia

Printed in Poland by Białostockie Zakłady Graficzne SA

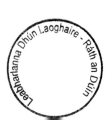

Contents

On Dominic

It's 2006 and I'm hobbling around JFK airport two days after running the marathon in NYC and I realise I have forgotten to book a flight ticket for my wife so that we could fly to Miami and start our honeymoon. She retells this story many times and who could blame her? In 2005, I had agreed to train a group of people to take on the challenge of running the New York marathon. I had met Gráinne by then, on a blind date, but the thing I didn't know was that by the time of the marathon, we'd be two weeks married.

To say that I was sporty as a kid growing up in Newbridge, County Kildare, is an understatement. I played any sports that were available to me but the ones I enjoyed the most were athletics and basketball. The former taught me the importance to success of individual discipline and the latter gave me valuable insights into teamwork, comradery and unity. I kind of fell into doing Physiology and Health Sciences in Carlow RTC, simply because it sounded close to Sports Science or PE teaching, which I didn't have the smarts to get into at that time.

After two years spent in the midlands of Ireland I took the boat over to England to get my degree in Sports Science at the University of Sunderland. This wasn't the idyllic England as seen on the *Antiques Roadshow*. It was working class, mostly rainy and, although it gave me a brilliant education and social life, it also hardened me to the realities of life.

After my degree, I returned to Ireland and spent my early twenties working for a large commercial gym but, year by year, I got beaten down from teaching too many spinning and group exercise classes. I left the booming gym scene exhausted but determined to set up my own personal training business because waking up feeling wrong about having to train people in a way I knew wasn't optimal was killing me. I had years of practical experience in everything from Ashtanga yoga to weight training and had moulded a range of training methods into my way. I had no clients and no base to train from when I met Lisa Fitzpatrick. She became one of my first clients. She also owned a hairdresser's in Foxrock village and I spent many a Saturday sitting in her hair salon chatting with potential and future clients of mine, giving advice on nutrition and training. This developed into a thriving business and Lisa also set me up on a blind date with my future wife, Gráinne, when I thought I was just meeting another potential client. I invited her over for dinner and despite asking her ridiculous questions like 'what are the last five books you read', I sparked enough interest to secure a second date.

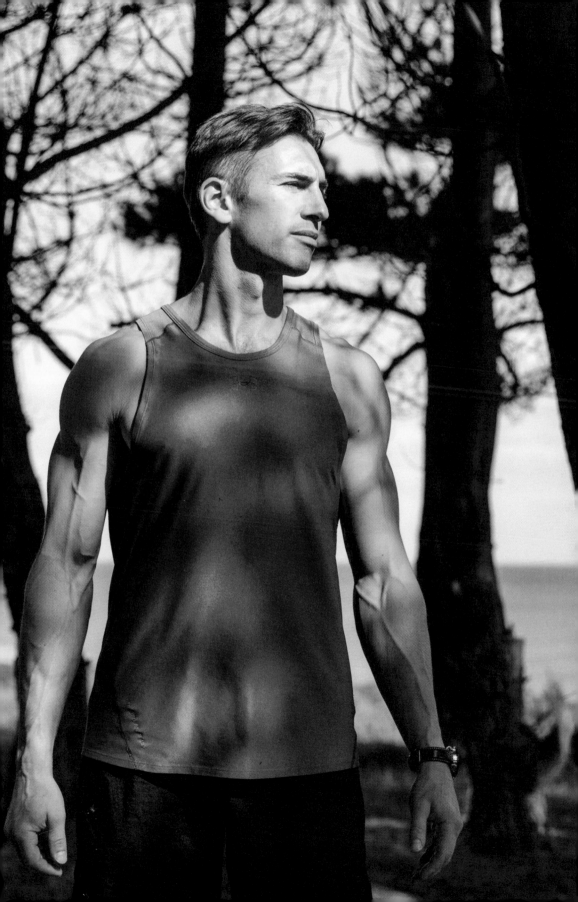

Obsession is a curse and a gift. My dedication to further education and training had left me very well educated and in great shape but I lacked the emotional intelligence needed to give my life true balance. Gráinne gave me that through her appreciation and love of *la dolce vita*, as she had just returned from a long career break in Italy and was rekindling her love of cooking and yoga. Many a Sunday was filled with yoga classes and a trip to the farmers' market. My nutrition was always about exclusion (gluten free, dairy free, flavour free!); that radically changed to what I needed to include. My health compulsion had even extended to praising the merits of chicory-root coffee. Gráinne showed me the error of my ways by introducing me to properly made delectable coffee long before the hipster coffee boom in Dublin. Fast forward more than ten years later, to a wonderful daughter and a life that has not been easy to balance; yet we've remained steadfast in our love of the benefits of good food and regular exercise and try to pass on those values to our growing child. They say that behind every great man is a woman, but she's beside him and with him, not behind him. Gráinne has been beside me and supported me every step of the way. I hope you take from this book our combined and unified approach to fitness, health and wellness to give you the best possible approach to training and treating your body the way nature intended.

On Gráinne

By the time I was 32 I had buried my first husband after his sudden death on a mountain in France. It is that horrific event which brought me to where I am today.

I have always cooked – my earliest memories are of making brown and white soda bread, graduating from being allowed only to cut the cross to eventually being trusted to make the whole thing. Then learning to make pastry and discovering I had 'cold hands', which are apparently the best hands for making pastry. I used to love Saturday nights if mum and dad went out: finally, I had the kitchen to myself – mum said she used to wonder what the state of the kitchen would be when they got home but that at least there would be something to offer if people came in for a drink after a night out.

As the eldest girl and second eldest of six kids, cooking was helping but it was also something I enjoyed. I loved making cakes and there was a time when a chocolate chequerboard cake was my *pièce de résistance* though there was also a cat cake period (with spaghetti for whiskers) for my little sisters' parties. I have always liked to feed people and I got that from my mum – no matter how many people appeared, she didn't mind feeding them. When we were older, Sunday dinners usually featured boyfriends and girlfriends around the table as well as her own big gang.

I cooked through happy times and sad times and during those very sad times I think it probably kept me sane because when I cooked I was in the moment and, for that moment, my troubles melted away.

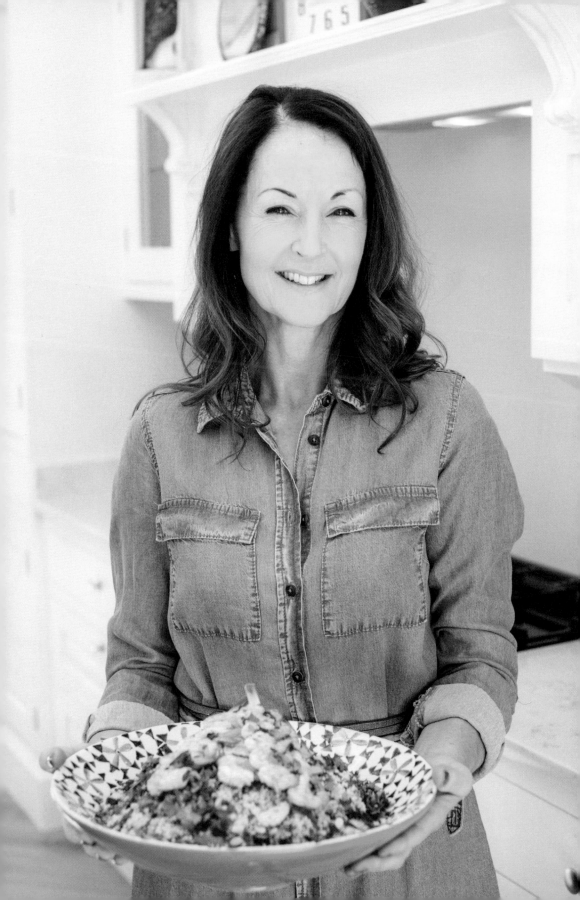

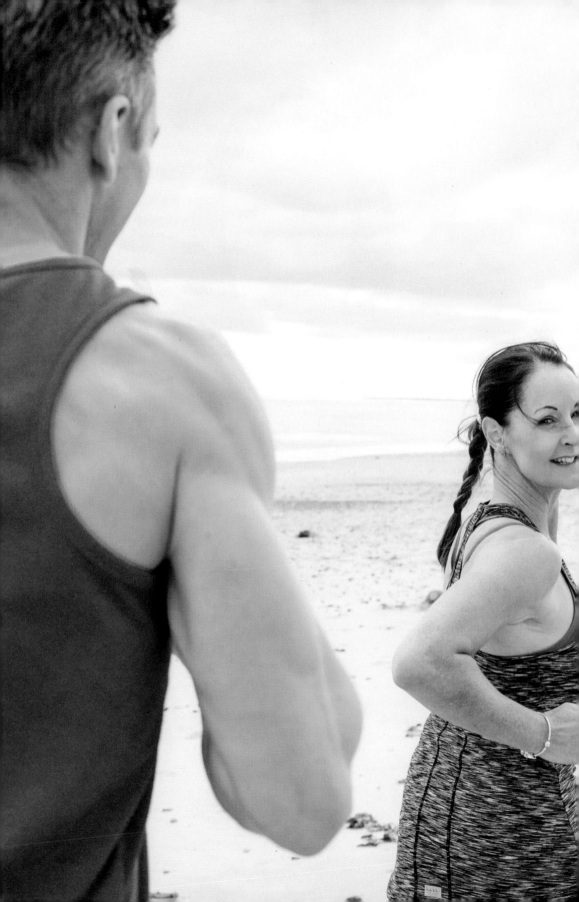

I was generally always active – when we were kids we were outside all day. I became mad about gymnastics and we used to practise morning, noon and night, outside in the garden or pushing the furniture back in the 'good' room to do our routines. I wasn't madly talented at any sport – I have loads of medals for the three-legged race on sports day and little else – but I was always strong and my brother talks about bringing his friends home from school to arm wrestle me because he used to make bets that I would beat them. Having played loads of sports all through school, I did what many girls do when I went to college and they mostly went out the window, apart from a little squash and tennis. Thankfully, I picked it back up and am so glad I did as being active does so much for my body and mind.

Life was happy and unremarkable until not quite two years into my first marriage, when my husband Ciárán died, the sadness and grief seemed unrelenting and unending. I hated to hear the clichés that 'Life goes on' and 'It will get easier' but eventually realised that it is sort of the truth. Eventually, a little light started to shine through (the cracks) and with it, I took up yoga, thanks to a suggestion from a friend at work, and found a connection again with my body and mind that helped the healing. After moving to Rome for time on my own, I returned to Ireland and, when I was ready, a blind date brought me Dominic and opened my life to love and happiness again as well as what being fit and strong really meant, way beyond any notions I might have had (lifting weights doesn't make you big) and, since I loved food and knew how to eat well, we were a marriage made in heaven. And while anyone who experiences loss will tell you that the scars are always there, being married to Dominic and having our daughter has brought me love, peace, happiness and has literally transformed my life. I am happy, fit and healthy. I have stepped away from a very busy career in consulting because I want to show people how it is possible to be all those things and work or have a family or both. I'm 25 years old in my head and, while in reality I am much more than that, being fit and healthy means that at 50+, I can do a handstand and lift weights and that makes me proud of my body and all it can achieve. I went back to study health and wellness coaching because I would like to be able to help people achieve their most cherished health and wellness goals and live fit, happy and healthy lives, like we were meant to.

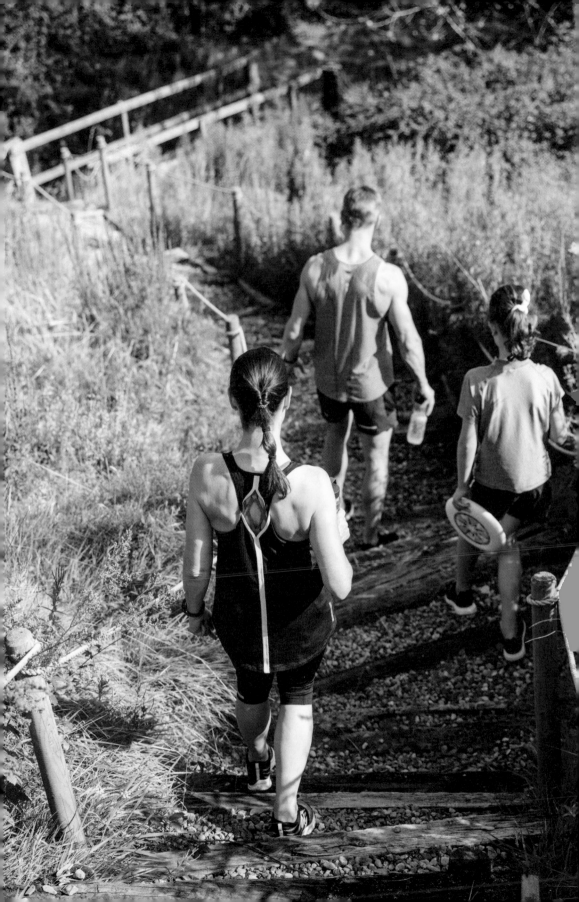

What's in this book and how to use it

This book incorporates the experience we have gleaned from 20 years of working with clients, helping them feel better, fitter, healthier and happier. Here you will learn why and how to develop your flexibility as the foundation to being fit and why it should be your priority before addressing conditioning and strength. In our Train Well chapter you will learn why you should listen to and understand how your body is feeling before you train and why beating yourself up in the gym will never deliver the results you would like. We show a sensible, more compassionate approach to becoming fit. We teach you the fundamentals of good nutrition and how to bring awareness to what you eat so that you can lose the weight you want and eat better for life. Our recipes are healthy, calorie-counted and tailor-made for the whole family. Our Being Well chapter brings being well to the forefront with strategies to help you improve your sleep, develop resilience to stress and be happier. This book encompasses everything you need to learn to be a fitter, healthier, happier you.

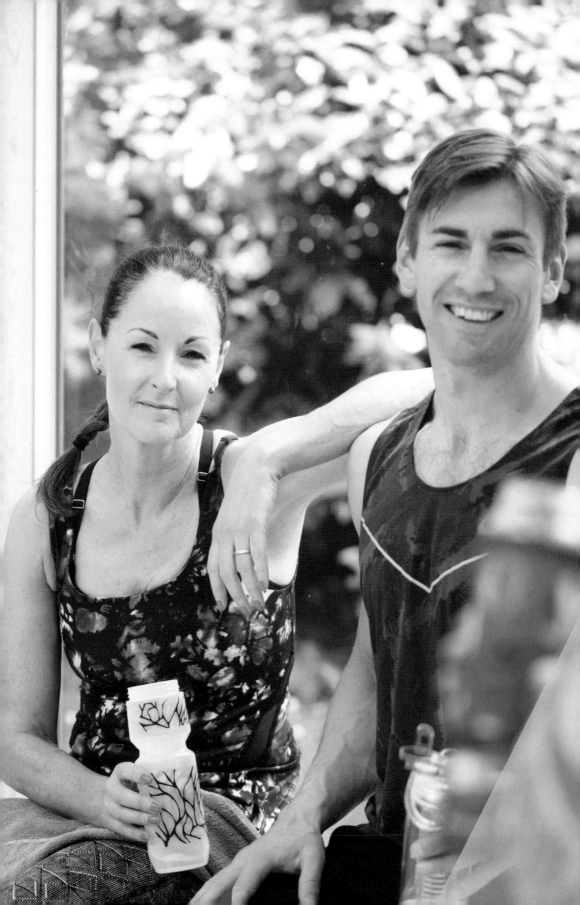

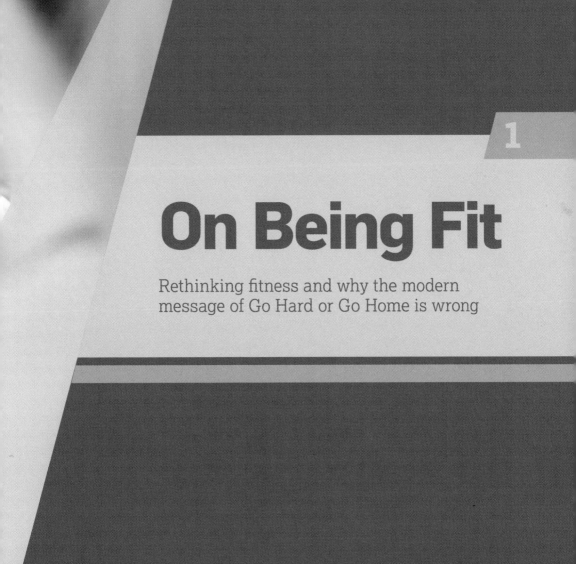

1

On Being Fit

Rethinking fitness and why the modern
message of Go Hard or Go Home is wrong

This book is for you.

This is the book I wish I'd had when I first started training and working with clients many years ago.

Climbing trees, running, jumping, skipping, pretending I was the Karate Kid and playing a wide range of sports was how I spent my highly active youth. I look back on those times when, in fits of excitement, games of rounders were organised with neighbours and it gives me the opportunity to remember effortless movement and play.

There was no struggle in getting up off the floor, our energy was boundless and our hearts warmed to the simple pleasures we got from activities we have formalised into exercise.

Years spent in college gave me the science but as a trainee I was put to work in a commercial gym and indoctrinated into a way to approach exercise and training that was isolated and not integrated. In one corner, you had the cardio bunnies sweating away on the treadmills and cross trainers, the bodybuilders stuck to the section that had the most mirrors and those interested in yoga or flexibility were often seen as taking the easy way out. There was no cross-pollination of ideas because you were told they were separate goals.

Feeling exhausted and burnt-out from teaching too many classes forced me to find a better way to address how to train myself and clients. This was no easy task as I was wrapped up in an industry that was more focused on how many calories you burned, how intense your sessions were and how you looked.

A quote from Bruce Lee always stuck with me and directed me to form my own way to optimise health and fitness because what I was doing and what I was observing was limited and making me feel worse, not better.

> *Adapt what is useful, reject what is useless, and add what is specifically your own.*
>
> **Bruce Lee,**
> ***Tao of Jeet Kune Do* (1975)**

During the process of forming my own way of answering the question of what fitness is, I met and married my wife, we have a wonderful daughter now and they bring vital ingredients to the mix that I was definitely missing – a more compassionate, less restrictive point of view and a clear understanding of what's important in life. Tragedy, failure and joy are the greatest teachers and have given us many life lessons that allow us to speak from a place of experience and earned wisdom.

We're going to show and teach you why your understanding of fitness and the fitness industry's general promotion and approach to helping you feel and look better are incomplete. We want to give you advice that has stood the test of time and is relevant for you, no matter your age or your life circumstances.

Years spent helping clients feel and look their best has given us clearly defined principles to work from. We have never had to adjust our message according to trends; we focus on teaching and helping people remember how their body is intended to move and feel, using properly applied movement and nutrition. Modern life is busy and fast-paced; endless sitting, combined with a poor diet and inactivity,

'It is a shame for a man to grow old without seeing the beauty and strength of which his body is capable.'

Socrates

can lock us in to bad posture, feelings of constant tiredness, and weight gain. Moving well, feeling well and thinking well are all taken away from us in time from either lack of use or abuse. Health and fitness are a wonderful gift for those of us lucky enough to be born with them but you often don't appreciate something until it's gone. This is a book devoid of four-week quick fixes, 1,000-calorie macrobiotic diets, hacks to drop body fat or a dogmatic approach to nutrition. This is a user manual for your body that has its source firmly planted in 20 years of practical experience, consistently working with clients looking to lose weight, tone up, feel happier and thrive in a busy and stressful workplace environment.

It is a shame for a man to grow old without seeing the beauty and strength of which his body is capable.

Socrates

I came to realise that every activity is made more difficult with muscles that are stiff and tight, getting stronger is important up until a point and elevating your heart rate is great but making every workout into a heart-thumping maximal effort is a big mistake. What was I to do with an increasing number of clients who were practising fitness yet felt anything but fit? Add to that the people who were not coming because it all felt too confusing and too hard even to get started.

Origins of fitness and where it all went wrong

The body we have today has been moulded over thousands of years from basic functional movements that were required just to survive. We needed to sprint to catch food, or trek for hours, pick up objects to build homes and climb trees to avoid prey or enemies. In reality, nobody invented exercises like the deadlift because that's a movement we did throughout the ages to pick heavy objects off the floor. We didn't create the squat either; this is a movement that still exists today as a resting position for many cultures but the benefits have been lost to most of us from inactivity and sitting excessively in chairs due to most modern work. We possess a body that's been shaped by nature but that's not how we're using it.

We have changed how we move gradually in the last hundred years but we've drastically changed how we eat in the past 20 to 30 years.

If you were a child of the 1970s or 1980s you simply didn't have access to too many junk foods because they were not regularly bought. Your parents couldn't afford junk foods because they were luxury items that were only bought on rare occasions. If you were lucky and there was a family with a bit more money on your road then you looked forward to babysitting for them, not because their kids were easy to put to bed but because they had a filled biscuit tin and a soda stream.

Increased access and affordability have turned junk food into not only a daily option but a choice that's often cheaper than the healthier alternative. Fast forward 10 to 20 years and we see families buying half their food from a petrol station or local takeaway or shopping trolleys filled with boxed convenience food instead of

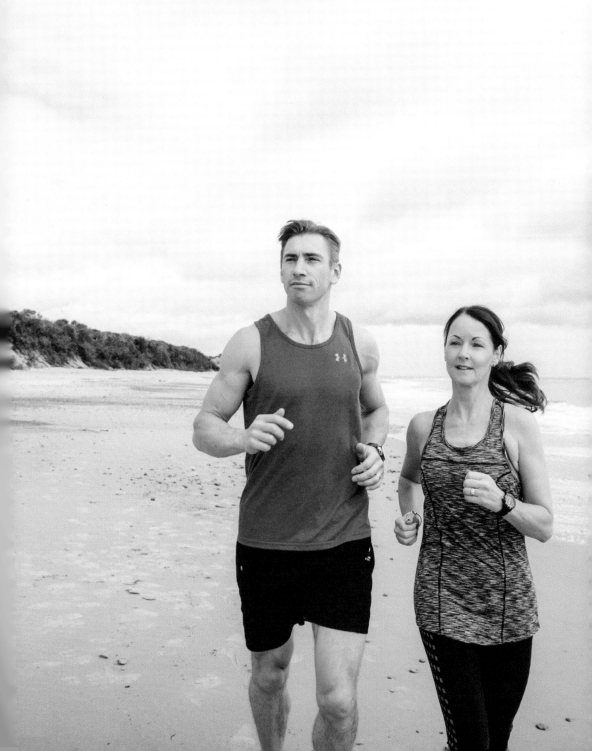

ingredients to make meals from scratch and sitting down to eat at a table. Our busy lives and increasingly longer working days have not helped but the truth is that we have moved too far away from the way we are meant to eat.

Eating well isn't a punishment, although people often start out thinking that it will be. Eating well means eating the food our body needs and likes; the flavours and tastes from properly cooked meat, fish, fruit and vegetables are just amazing, and not something to groan at the idea of.

Fitness has suffered the same commercialisation. It's bigger, stronger, faster all the way. One can no longer aspire simply to run a 5km or 10km race. Now you can't truly claim to be fit unless you've done an ultra-marathon (50km+ race), an ironman or, better still, do either in extreme weather conditions, such as the Marathon des Sables, a six-day ultramarathon held annually in the Sahara Desert. Remember, folks – no pain, no gain.

The bright colours and tight clothes from aerobics classes of the 1970s and 1980s have remained but dancing around the studio has been thrown out and we now have classes where intensity is key, such as Bootcamp, Inferno, Insanity, Body Attack, etc. We're constantly bombarded with the message that you need to work harder and that you are not getting results because you simply don't want it badly enough. This is one of the most damaging messages in fitness right now and it is causing many people to get over-trained, burnt out and injured.

> *How hard you train is never going to be as important as how consistently you train and too many people try to cure their lack of consistency with higher training intensity.*

We focus on teaching fitness as it applies to a body that has been shaped by natural movement and trained with periods of rest and recovery. The 'no pain, no gain' mantra needs to be replaced with 'training stress + rest = results'.

What is fitness?

When people talk about getting fit, they often think that the only thing they need to work on is their cardiorespiratory fitness because they feel a bit sluggish and think that if they get their heart rate up through running, for example, then that will demonstrate how fit they are.

There is no question whatsoever that elevating your breathing and heart rate will help build a stronger heart and more powerful lungs, which are vital for overall health and well-being but we want to be able to achieve this goal, and MORE, through the safest means possible. That is extremely challenging if the individual we are working with is not only unfit from a lungs-and-heart perspective but, more crucially, from a strength and flexibility perspective.

What is the use of being able to run 5k if you are so stiff you can't touch your toes and so weak you can't do a press-up. We address **ALL** aspects of fitness so that you can move without pain and be strong well into your old age.

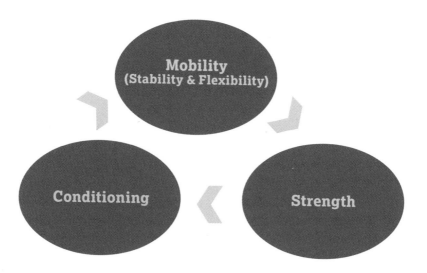

Fundamentals of Fitness

The model we present for what it means to be fit incorporates **ALL** aspects of fitness, such as flexibility, strength, speed, power, co-ordination, aerobic conditioning and anaerobic conditioning.

Mobility – the forgotten cornerstone of fitness

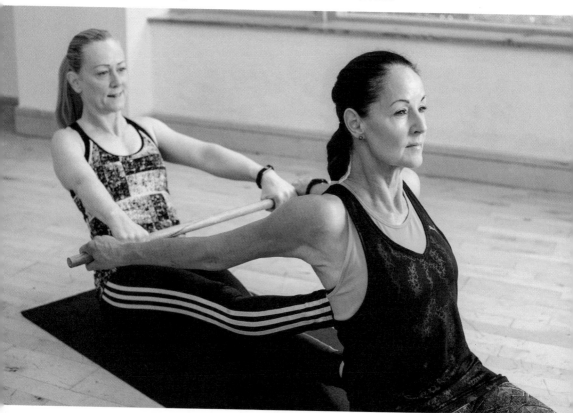

The top priority for everyone, and our foundation of fitness, is to be mobile. This means how well you move about, doing basic day-to-day activities pain-free and demonstrating passable levels of both stability and flexibility. This is because **stronger and more flexible muscles will make short work of ANY activity than smaller, tighter and weaker muscles**.

> *Mobility is a factor of both your ability to stabilise your muscles and your flexibility.*

You wouldn't drive your car with the handbrake on all the time but that is exactly what happens when you exercise or even just go about your day when your muscles are tight. If they're tight, they're also generally weak. In the next chapter, we will discuss mobility and some specific tests you can easily perform to check your level of mobility but a simple test you can perform easily to assess your mobility is the **'sitting-rising test'**.[1]

In a study on mobility and its link to mortality, physicians in Brazil came up with this quick test to measure your mobility:

The study found that the more often you needed to use your hands and knees the higher your mortality from all causes. This is a remarkable conclusion because it is the first time that muscle strength and flexibility have been linked to longevity.

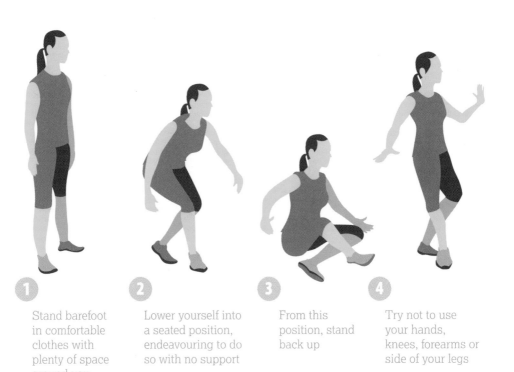

1 Stand barefoot in comfortable clothes with plenty of space around you

2 Lower yourself into a seated position, endeavouring to do so with no support

3 From this position, stand back up

4 Try not to use your hands, knees, forearms or side of your legs

We don't intend to scare you with this statement and obviously all of us are mortal in the end; however, understand that the more mobile we are, the better our movement quality is maintained into our older years. We are less likely to suffer trips or accidental falls, and daily activity is far easier.

If you're below 40 reading this, you may think 'Well, I'm not in my 60s so that doesn't concern me' but we run this test with clients all the time who are in their teens, 20s and 30s and many of them really struggle to get up and down without using their hands or knees. This is a major problem because if your mobility is poor at an early age it will only get progressively worse unless you realise how critical it really is to overall fitness. In addition, you're more likely to get injured and just feel stiff and sore all the time.

The typical markers of health have tended to be body mass index, blood pressure, cholesterol and blood glucose levels and, indeed, they are still valid, but the real importance of this study is that it shows there is a direct correlation between how physically strong and flexible you are and your lifespan. The recognition of this link is a positive development because it confirms what we would like **YOU** to focus on and forms the foundation of **OUR** fundamentals of fitness.

If your mobility is poor then trying to layer on conditioning without addressing the faulty movement mechanics arising from your poor mobility will decrease the effectiveness of your efforts to get fit.

It is very challenging to perform any basic activity properly with a body that is weak and tight. Yes, it is important to exercise regularly but the risk of injuring yourself in any form of exercise is higher if you are not addressing your poor mobility and strength. Exercise with a strong and flexible body is more enjoyable because your movement quality is optimal and all the right muscles can work effectively and take the appropriate loading in the right way. The fitness industry has made us more aware of exercise to improve our conditioning but in general does a terrible job of addressing mobility. Evidence of this is the high rate of injuries among the gym or exercising population.

> *Basic mobility is not a choice: it's a must-have aspect of your fitness that needs to be developed and is covered comprehensively in this book.*

Strength

The second layer to our fitness model is to build and maintain strength. Strength is your ability to carry and move your own body in day-to-day activity and in performing basic primal movements, such as the squat, deadlift, push-up and pull-up, and midline stability (strong core muscles). Modern life has us spending more time sitting than ever before and this causes huge and sometimes irreversible changes in our bodies. Hours in work hunched over a desk is generally followed by more time after work spent slouched on a sofa. This weakens our muscles which makes it harder to perform hardwired movements we could do with ease as a child.

Maintaining and building strength at all ages is vital to overall health, as it aids in:

- Increasing metabolism
- Promoting fat loss
- Improved balance and co-ordination
- Improved muscular tone
- Improved blood glucose control
- Boosting confidence through feeling good from exercise and better body image

All the benefits of strength training can be achieved by using your own body weight or external tools, such as bands, dumb-bells or kettlebells to provide a resistance for your muscles to work against. The tools you use to build strength are largely irrelevant as all your body knows is that it's being asked to work against a force and it must adapt to the stress it's being put under. The fitness industry loves to sell us the idea that a fancy new exercise tool or machine is going to give you better results, yet **the most important aspect of training is not the tools you pick but the consistency at which you train**.

Where are all the vibration plates, the abdominal crunchers and thigh-masters? On the scrapheap along with the hopes and dreams of the people that bought them. Buying fitness equipment became a national pastime. Don't make that mistake. Instead, stick to what has worked for decades and what is going to continue to work for years to come. The movements that will give you the biggest bang for your buck are basic and can be performed with little or no equipment.

Strength training as promoted by much of the fitness industry tends to be badly explained and demonstrated poorly. Strength training sold as exercises done only for high repetitions (or reps), with a disregard for movement, form or technique and no training principles other than to push hard and do more, is not sustainable and will lead to injury and a plateau in progress.

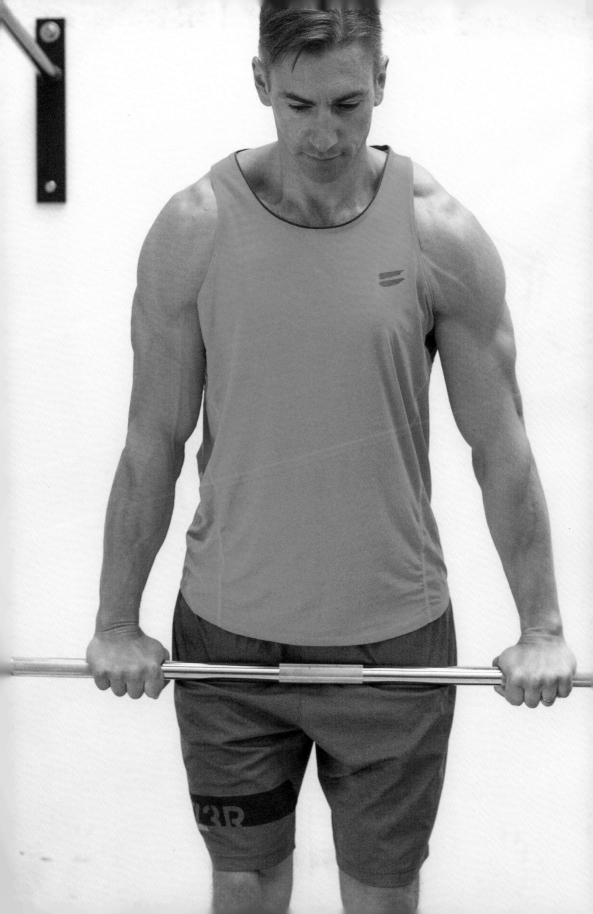

To develop usable strength, you should follow these four principles:

1. **Use multi-joint movements** – a squat will work more muscles than a leg-extension machine; a deadlift will deliver more than doing seven different glute or butt exercises. We don't need to be performing twelve different exercises in each training session: we just need to do the simple movements well.

2. **Reps, reps, reps** – just like learning any new skill, you must practise, practise, practise. Doing the movements often will build muscle and strength but how hard you push it needs to be moderated as doing too much can hinder progress. Your body has a limited capacity to recover from workouts and this varies from one person to the next. The general rule should be to listen to your body. Observe and feel how you're moving on the day. If you are doing your warm-up and feel like you have plenty of energy and pep, then push harder on that day, but if everything feels sluggish, you slept badly and just don't feel that good, then that's a day to pull back and lower the intensity and loading on all movements. It's not being lazy, but being sensible and kind to yourself.

3. **Variety** – you can change how you do the basic movements quite easily and this sends a signal to your body to adapt to a different stimulus. This can be done through changing the speed of the repetitions you do, the load used, the tool used (kettlebell/dumb-bell/bands, etc.) and how it is held.

4. **Progressive resistance** – you might have been told in the past that using some light water bottles will help you get in shape. All you need is to jump around your living room with body-weight movements. This may very well be a great starting point for some people but in order to get stronger you need to, well, get stronger! There's a point where using a water bottle as an external resistance is not enough because muscles need enough stimulation or overload. We don't mean lifting very heavy weights – we're big believers in there being a point where 'strong' is 'strong enough', but you will need to build some basic competency in functional movements before this is ever the case. I have heard time and time again, 'I don't want to get too big', and my answer is that it won't happen overnight; you will know when you are strong enough and look and feel the way you want to. It is also relative to where your mobility is limiting you, i.e. if you're very tight then pushing the strength numbers should take a back seat until the mobility catches up.

Some basic strength standards we would like to see are listed below but keep in mind that these might be very long- or short-term goals, depending your starting point:

- Push-ups and pull-ups with your own body weight for a rep or multiple reps;
- Deadlift and squat your own body weight e.g. if you're a 60kg woman then you should be eventually able to lift 50–60kg on your back in a squat, or off the floor in a deadlift;

- Complete our core test: ability to hold a hollow body shape for 30 seconds with feet 15–30 cm off the floor or 30 seconds holding a toes-pointed plank position.

Working on these goals will provide you with an excellent strength base that will make all activities far easier. There are, of course, exceptions to the above: you may have a long-standing injury or mechanical issue that can make some of these movements impossible for you, but there are always ways to scale and adjust movements to where you're limited so you too can benefit from getting stronger.

Conditioning

The last element we need for optimal fitness is conditioning and this is often the most abused. Conditioning can be broken into two main areas – aerobic fitness and anaerobic fitness.

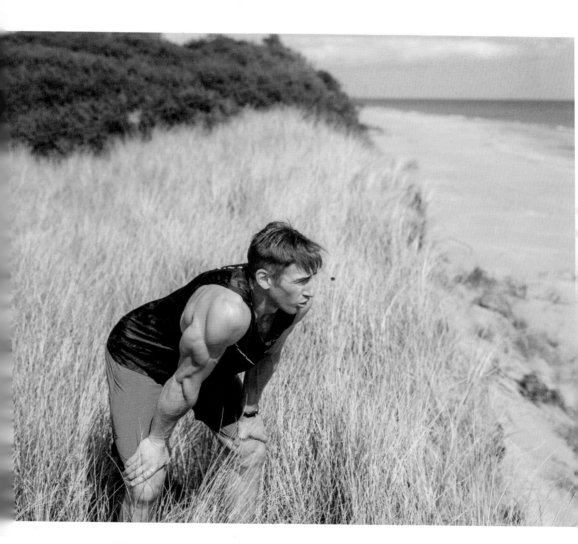

Aerobic fitness – your ability to maintain a low heart rate for a long period of time; improves the body's cardiovascular efficiency and cellular energy is produced with the use of oxygen. Working on this type of fitness should feel easy and must be done at a steady pace.

Anaerobic fitness – your capacity to handle short, hard bursts of activity; improves the body's cardiovascular efficiency and cellular energy is produced without the use of oxygen. Working on this type of fitness will feel very challenging and is typically done at a fast pace.

This is an important distinction to understand because conditioning must be built through an aerobic fitness base first and a gradual introduction to anaerobic fitness second. You won't be able to handle higher-intensity work if you have not built a base of lower-intensity work initially. The higher the intensity of exercise or work performed, the more stressful it is to your body and the longer it takes to recover from.

We frequently work with clients who jumped straight into harder and more intense exercise, which is a problem because they had not built the base that helps and teaches your body to handle or buffer byproducts of exercise, such as lactic acid. Think of a tap you have running very slowly and then you open it up fully so that water is pouring out uncontrollably. This is what happens to someone with no aerobic base who tries to exercise too hard too often: they are turning that tap on full power all the time, which is unsustainable and can lead to burnout and injuries.

There has been a big push in the past five to ten years towards high-intensity interval training.[2] This is mainly due to the numerous scientific studies that have shown that short bursts of high-intensity exercise, e.g. riding an exercise bike hard for 20 seconds, recovering by cycling slowly for 90–120 seconds and repeating three to five times, can elicit the same cardiorespiratory and blood glucose control benefits as moderate exercise for 30–45 minutes. This leads to attractive headlines, such as 'One minute of all-out exercise may have benefits of 45 minutes of moderate exertion.' There's also the promise or hope that harder workouts burn more fat than lower-intensity workouts.

However, what we find in practice is that exposing clients to very high intensity increases risk of injury. Firstly, it is not practical for those already carrying injuries. Secondly, we have observed more muscle tears, falls and trips as a direct result of high-intensity work. You can't exercise if you are injured or sick. Also if you want to do higher-intensity exercise you must earn the right to go hard by having a body that's both mobile and strong enough to handle it.

Build a base at moderate levels first. To develop that base, you must firstly have the capacity to work continually for 30–60 minutes without getting exhausted.

Mary's Story

Mary needs to lose weight and hasn't been exercising in quite a while. Any activity is going to increase her heart rate and if pushed too much she will tip over from aerobic into anaerobic fitness. The solution is to build up her conditioning primarily through low-intensity sessions and have no more than one session per week where we push the intensity for a short duration, e.g. some interval work of high and low intensity performed on a low-impact piece of equipment, such as exercise bike, rower, cross trainer or sled push.

Low-intensity sessions should be a mixture of mobility, strength and conditioning work, with the aim of keeping everything lower than six out of ten (where ten is maximum effort) because even the act of working on simple things like stretching and foam rolling (see page 31) is going to feel like hard work for someone with no exercise history. Added weight will make all activities more challenging. Mary will often have huge gaps in her mobility and strength so this approach is an excellent way to address all aspects of her fitness.

We already have more than enough stress being layered on us through work and life so the last thing someone who is new to exercise needs is to be pushed to their limits.

Low-intensity sessions with a bias towards more mobility, some strength and a little bit of conditioning are also something you should do if you are feeling tired, carrying an injury or just have a lot going on in life. The more you push yourself the more cortisol you produce. Cortisol is a stress hormone that isn't harmful when produced in low amounts but can be devastating if you are pumping it out from training sessions that are too high in intensity and then combining that with poor nutrition, lack of sleep and other external life stressors. We all have a limit in our ability to recover, so learn to know your limits. Exercise often but get better at knowing when to push and when to hold back.

How we get you fit

A breakdown of a typical week for the average person might look like the following:

- Mobility work performed daily for 15–20 minutes
- Our workouts, performed three to five times per week
- After three to four weeks of building an aerobic base, improving mobility and strength, introduce one session per week of higher intensity (i.e. push yourself harder)

'Any fool can create a program that is so demanding that it would virtually kill the toughest Marine or hardiest of elite athletes. But not any fool can create a tough program that produces progress without unnecessary pain.'

**Dr Mel C. Siff –
author of *Supertraining***

We all have much the same body that needs to be trained by building fitness through principled methods rather than by throwing a bunch of movements into a bowl, stirring it up and praying something will work. Some people would argue that that is better than nothing. It's not if it's causing you to get injured or not addressing where you need to work on physically.

We have spent over 20 years testing, checking, assessing and now presenting the best way to approach fitness and physical well-being so you don't need to search any more.

Only a fool learns from his own mistakes; a wise man learns from the mistakes of others.

Otto von Bismarck

This is fitness that is sustainable, practicable and principle-led vs quick fixes, promised rapid results and laden with risk.

Am I too old for this?

Fitness is neatly sold to us through exuberance, youth and inexperience and can leave many people feeling excluded. Many of the clients we've worked with for ten or more years and who started in their 40s or 50s admitted that if they had not got started at that age or stage in their life, they would have given up and felt it just wasn't for them. Fitness is a basic requirement for all ages and you should never be made to feel inadequate or excluded.

Most people will tell you as you grow older that you need to accept your ageing body, throw on the comfortable shoes and accept you will get man boobs. I urge you NOT to accept this as an inevitable part of getting older.

The Welsh poet Dylan Thomas wrote one of my favourite poems, 'Do not go gentle into that good night'. Its life-affirming line should spur you on to get up and act from where you are today: **'Old age should burn and rave at close of day; Rage, rage against the dying of the light.'**

Make changes now so that you don't have to accept your life with limits, medication and slippers. Make a decision – stay the same or make a change.

We will give you the tools throughout this book to feel your best so let's get started with assessing and helping you fix your mobility.

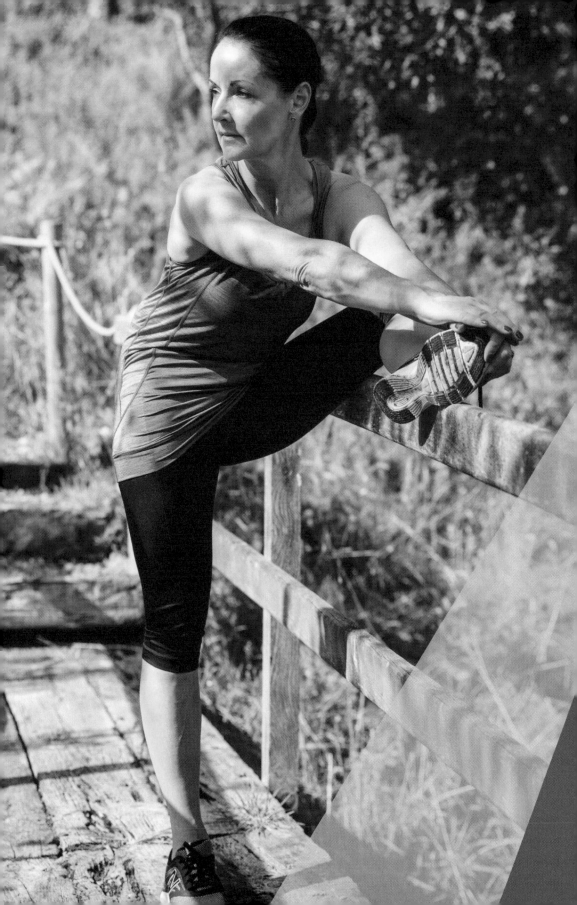

Your body knows functional movements like squats, pull-ups and deadlifts. It knows the best way to eat and be satisfied, knows how to sleep to feel fully rested, knows what it is like when it is happy after time spent with family or on your favourite hobby. It just needs to be reminded.

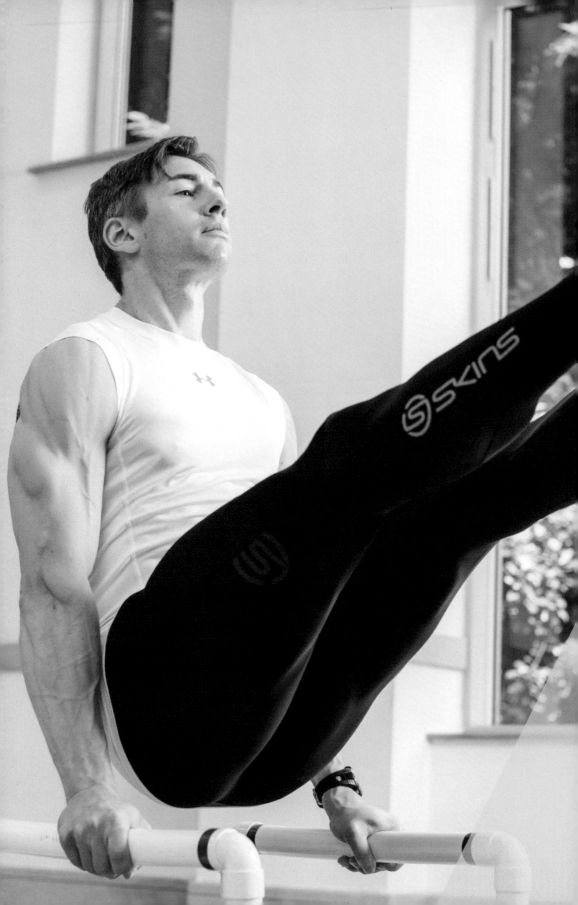

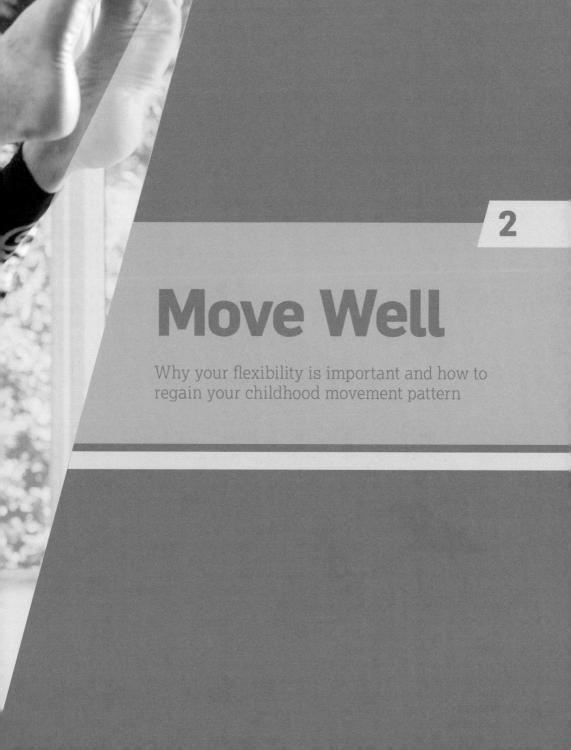

2

Move Well

Why your flexibility is important and how to
regain your childhood movement pattern

How to take the handbrake off

We believe it's easier to observe beautiful movement (define that as being mobile) and then work backwards from those who possess such qualities. *Adagio* is a ballet term that means 'at ease'. We appreciate the fluid movements of yoga, the controlled power of gymnastics, the pointed toes and grace of ballet and dance. When we look at the best movers in the world, they all have an ease to their performance. Keep these images in mind when you think about working on your mobility and how your body should feel most of the time; it should feel *adagio*.

Developing mobility is often seen as a passive activity that requires you to relax into it but that could not be further from the truth. It is one of the biggest misconceptions on how people who possess amazing mobility go about developing it.

When we have discussions around how to develop strength and conditioning, most people have a fair idea how to get started, yet mobility is always treated with mystery and boredom. Working on how well you move is not as cool and sexy as sweating and lifting weights yet it is essential if you want to feel fit and prevent injuries.

Unfortunately, of all the components of fitness, improving your mobility can take the longest due to muscles that have been allowed to grind to a halt from years of lack of use or overuse. You will always feel as old as how your body moves. This is not just related to age: I work with clients in their 60s and beyond who move well and are pain-free and clients in their teens and twenties who move poorly and pick up injuries all the time due to muscles that have been allowed to become weak and tight.

> *You wouldn't try to drive your car with the handbrake on but that's exactly what's happening when you try to perform any activity with muscles that are weak and tight.*

From the ground up

If we look at the body joint by joint from the ground up it will give us a better understanding as to how to address our mobility and what we need to actively work on daily.

Grey Cook[1] MSPT, OCS, CSCS is a practising physical therapist, an orthopaedic-certified specialist and a leading figure in the fitness and physical therapy industry. His approach on how to improve functional movement has been central to helping us understand mobility. He explains, if we look at the feet, that we want the arches to be stable but ankles to be mobile. From there we want the knees to be stable but the hips to be mobile and so it moves over and back between stability and mobility as we move up the chain.

If we use this as a template for understanding the body in movement, it's easier to be clear on what is causing the greatest disability worldwide: lower back pain.

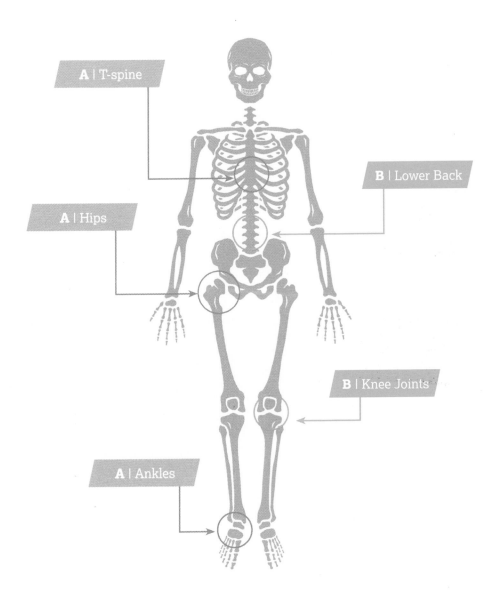

A | T-spine

B | Lower Back

A | Hips

B | Knee Joints

A | Ankles

A = Mobility
B = Stability

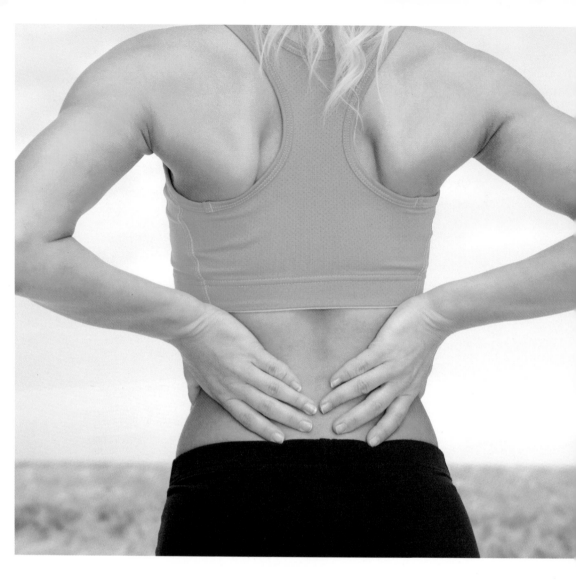

Studies have shown that higher-income countries have a two to four times higher rate of back pain compared to low-income countries. In less-developed countries people regularly carry heavy loads yet experience less back pain.

One of the main causes of lower back pain is the length of time people spend sitting in chairs without any type of activity at all. Excessive sitting causes areas that are supposed to be mobile to become stiff and weak (ankles, hips, thoracic spine) and the parts of your body that should be stable (feet, knees, lower back) get forced into becoming mobile. Sitting, however, does not apply to sitting on the floor where the hips, in particular, will open up more as they were naturally intended to and are not held in chronically tight positions. Sitting has been branded as the new smoking, with research papers and articles linking it to cancer, heart disease, diabetes and depression. There's an entire industry that's now dedicated to selling stand-up desks so you can do all or some of your work in a standing position to help mitigate the negative effects of sitting. While I don't believe we should put sitting in the same box as smoking, we definitely need to address it. We need to look at the context of sitting. Studies so far show that sitting down at work isn't strongly linked with long-term degenerative diseases, but sitting watching TV is consistently linked with increased mortality. Is this because those who watch more TV tend to be less active, and through watching TV are exposed to more advertising for junk foods or is it just from the negative effects of sitting? What we need to focus on is getting you moving well and often rather than turning sitting into a scapegoat for all our ailments.

The lower back largely becomes an issue because your hips, ankles and thoracic spine become chronically tight and you are then by default asking your lower back to become mobile. The problem with this is that the lower back is not designed for the mobility being requested of it and, as a result, it becomes aggravated and sore, yet the main driver of this issue is often tight hips, weak glutes and core.

Once pain is present, it becomes a driver of muscle tone and tension, compounding the problem with distorted motor control.[2]

Asking stable joints to work overtime can lead people into focusing on one area when it might not be the source of the pain.

Perry Nickelston, DC, NKT, FMS, SFMA is a Chiropractic Physician with a primary focus on performance enhancement and he is often quoted as saying:

Pain only tells you there's a problem, it does not tell you what it is. Very often pain is a compensation pattern.[3]

With the application of a joint-by-joint approach we develop a simple plan of action to work with when we start assessing and addressing our mobility because we now know which joints need to be mobile and which need to be stable. This helps us to target the right areas and prevent needless hammering away to relieve pain in, for example, the knee, when quite often it's tight hips and ankles combined with poor muscle strength around the knee joint that is the primary driver of the pain.

With any new client, we start by doing a mobility assessment. What we want from this is to check how well the mobile joints are moving and test how stable the stable areas really are. What we've discovered from doing this with hundreds of clients over the years is that lack of activity has made the hips, ankles and thoracic spine very tight and weak, which makes it harder to get fit because your body doesn't move how it should and this can increase the risk of injury.

This doesn't mean we spend hours and weeks doing rehabilitation sessions. What it does mean is that we devote time to addressing your mobility needs, based on how you perform on the following tests.

Assess and Improve Your Mobility

The first four test your flexibility or range of motion and the last tests core stability. Score yourself from 1-5 on each test, where 1 = this is impossible, 5 = no problem at all.

01 Shoulder Dislocate

This is used to check what your shoulder mobility is like.

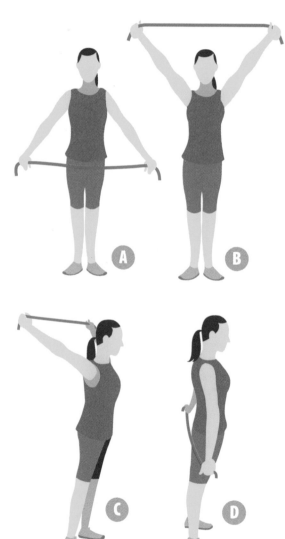

Using a broomstick or bands take a grip out in front of you about 15–30 cm wider than shoulder width. With arms held totally straight try to rotate the stick overhead and behind you right down to your bum.

If your arms bend at all, don't go beyond that point. If you can do this easily, then move the hands in slightly and go again until it is more challenging to pass through a 180-degree rotation of the arms. The shoulder blades should be pulled back and the chest pushed up throughout. Aim for ten reps slowly moving over and back, taking 5–10 seconds per rep.

Score: if you can't take the band or stick overhead and slightly behind you at all with straight arms, then score this as a 1; if you can pass over and back easily with a grip slightly wider than shoulder then score this as a 5.

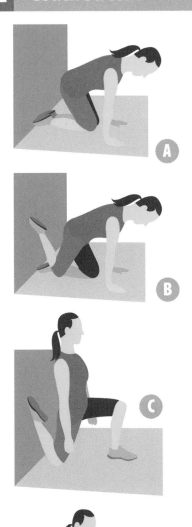

Get yourself next to a wall and kneel on all fours with feet very close to the wall and your body facing away from it. With hands still on the floor put your right knee on the floor a couple of centimetres away from the wall (closer shows better mobility) with the right leg now leaning against the wall and toes pointing towards the ceiling.

Step the left leg forwards so there is a 90-degree angle in the front left knee. Lift the chest up so you're in an upright position and try to put your back against the wall as you lie backwards into the wall.

You should feel a strong stretch in the hip flexors and thighs on the right leg. Repeat on opposite side. If you find this really difficult then move the knee that's close to the wall away from the wall a few centimetres until you can get the opposite leg at a 90-degree angle. Hold for 30–60 seconds per leg.

Score: 1 = you can't put you front foot out at all, 5 = you can put your upper back against the wall with the knee next to the wall.

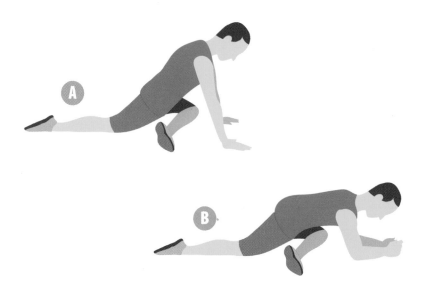

If you're very tight in this stretch and the previous one, it's quite likely you'll have back problems or knee problems due to lack of mobility.

To perform the stretch, get on all fours on the floor and bring the left knee to your left hand. As you do this, stretch the right leg out behind you. From there, lean slightly to the left and, using your right hand, pull the left foot forwards as much as it will go. The goal is to have the left foot in line with the left knee. Don't force it and only take it as high as it will go.

Your upper body should be leaning slightly to the right. Repeat on opposite side. Hold for 30–60 seconds per side to improve the stretch.

Score: 1 = the foot will not move up at all and is nowhere near being in line with the knee, 5 = foot is almost or is in line with the knee and your chest is flat to the floor as you lie over the front leg.

Single-leg Downward Dog Stretch

This is used to check what your calf and ankle mobility is like.

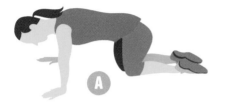

A

We see a strong connection between this stretch and how tight your hamstrings can get. Start on all fours again and lift knees off the floor. With hands and feet only on the floor, push your bum up into the air so you adopt a downward dog position that you typically see in yoga.

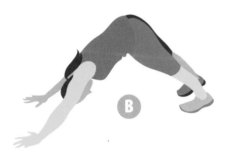

B

Drive your head through your arms so you're looking down towards your toes and then press your heels into the floor. While in this position, lift your right foot and put it behind the left foot so you use it to press the heel of the left foot into the floor. The left leg MUST remain straight.

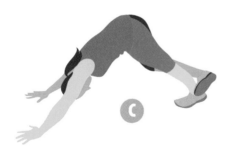

C

Repeat on opposite side. Hold for 30–60 seconds per side.

Score – 1 = heel of the straight leg is more than 3–5 centimetres off the floor, 5 = you can press both feet flat on the floor with head through the arms.

05 | Hollow Hold Core Test

This is used to check how stable you are. One of the main areas of instability in people is their core or midline.

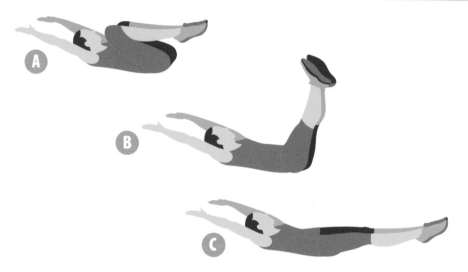

To do the test lie on your back with knees bent and feet on the floor. Straighten the arms out behind you. Lift your feet off the floor, press the lower part of the back into the floor by contracting the abdominal muscles hard. As you do so, lift the chest towards the ceiling so the head and top of shoulders are off the floor.

The arms are still totally straight and almost touching your ears. From there, straighten the legs as much as you can so your toes point towards the ceiling. The lower part of the back MUST remain in contact with the floor as you now start to move the straight legs very slowly towards the floor. The goal is to have the feet almost touching the floor with pointed toes and having no arch in the lower part of the back. Lower back is pressed into the floor.

Hold whatever position has you working hard to keep the arch out of the lower part of your back as you contract the abdominal muscles hard to do so and constantly keeping your pelvis tilted backwards.

Hold for 20–30 seconds.

Score: 1 = legs are bent and it is a struggle to point them towards the ceiling; 5 = legs perfectly straight with feet a few centimetres off the floor.

Give yourself a rough score on all five tests and keep in mind that a perfect score of 25 does not represent exceptional mobility, but shows normal ranges of motion. If your combined score is below 15 then you should be giving over at least 50 per cent of all training time to working on mobility.

The five tests shown are the most important movements you need to do daily. They should be combined with some self-massage methods, such as foam rolling.

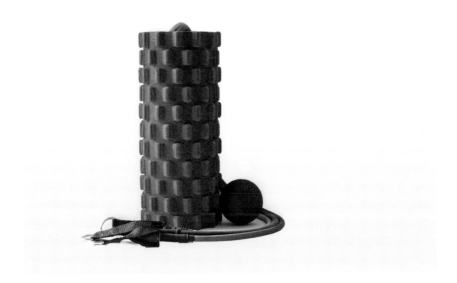

Pictured above is the typical equipment we use to help improve mobility. They include bands, foam rollers and balls, and we cover these below.

Rolling is typically done using a 61cm cylinder that is covered in a soft foam, or using a hard rubber ball, such as a lacrosse ball. You can pick up a foam roll in any sports store, or in some of the supermarket chains, which stock them from time to time.

The purpose of foam rolling is to help to loosen muscle tissue and improve its quality so that when you stretch it feels a little easier. It's a bit like someone giving you a massage and working on areas that you're tight in. The foam roll is normally best applied to the big muscle groups – thighs, hamstrings, upper back, calves, etc. – and the ball can be used for the hard-to-get-at areas that require the pressure to be a little more focused, such as glutes, rotator cuff in shoulders, forearms, plantar flexors on the base of your feet, etc.

Foam rolling will NOT significantly improve your mobility unless combined with stretching. There has been a trend over the past five to ten years of people spending far too much time rolling instead of using it as preparation for stretching. Stretching will make a more significant and lasting effect on your mobility so do some rolling but don't become that person who falls in love with their foam roll yet still can't score well on the mobility tests covered previously.

For some people, there are certain areas that become particularly stuck and no amount of self-massage and stretching help, so it is good to work with someone to help loosen out these areas, such as a physiotherapist, physical therapist or osteopath. I have often found that a few sessions with a specialist can help the client make big leaps in very tight areas to the point where they can manage their mobility themselves. The goal is to learn where you're tight/weak and know how to treat these areas yourself BEFORE they become major limitations.

After we have gone through the tests with a client, we take them through an active warm-up where we combine the previous tests done as mobility work paired with something to increase their body temperature, for example, one minute of light rowing, jogging, pushing a sled, stationary bike work, etc., and some band work.

Bands are an excellent tool for activating areas that need to be firing properly when training. The areas we tend to spend the most amount of time working on with clients are:

1. **Upper back** – most people have tight and rounded shoulders so warm them up with shoulder shrugs, moving the shoulders up to the ears and back; arm swings, where you rotate your arm around in a circle going forwards and backwards in turn; using the band to perform band pull-aparts where you hold the ends of the band in each hand and stretch the band apart to warm up the shoulders; and some shoulder dislocates as shown previously.

2. **Glutes** – if these muscles are not firing right then we need to liven them up with some X-band walks, where you take the band and place both feet on it while holding on to it with your hands. Now switch the grips of your hands so the band forms the appearance of an X. Walk sideways by stepping your right leg out and, when it contacts the ground, bring your left leg towards it but keep your feet shoulder-width apart. If you do this movement ten steps out and ten steps back for a few rounds it will really help the glutes fire.

We typically spend about ten minutes with clients doing a circuit of band work, cardio, foam rolling and mobility drills.

Note: Your mobility can often vary wildly depending on how active or inactive you've been in the last year. If you play a sport or perform an activity you're not used to, this can lead to stiff and sore muscles the next day. The same is true if you have been inactive from long-distance driving, working long hours at a desk, or even from poor nutrition and insufficient sleep. When we work with new or existing clients we will always perform a warm-up that allows us check how you are moving and then adjust the training session according to what is presented. If you feel you're very tight, don't be afraid to give over more of the training session to mobility work or even to make the entire session an extended warm-up. We firmly believe that everyone needs to spend one entire week in every six focusing significantly on mobility. If it is not done, what we often see is muscle stiffness and weakness creeping back in, thus making injuries more likely.

Breathing

The final element to taking the handbrake off is taking advantage of the power of your breath.

We all know the power of eating right towards helping us look and feel our best, but one of the most undervalued practices, and one which we can develop daily, is to learn how to use our breath to help relieve stress and to help prevent injuries.

Very few people know how to breathe correctly. Now I know what you're thinking: 'But I'm breathing ALL the time, so I wouldn't be alive if I wasn't doing it right!' Of course, you're going to be breathing but we want you to breathe efficiently so you can benefit from both its calming and bracing effects.

When you breathe, you should be using your diaphragm, the big dome-shaped muscle below the ribcage. How to test if you are using your diaphragm is to lie on your back with your feet against a wall or up on a bench/chair with the knees at a 90-degree angle. From there, take a big breath in and notice if your stomach moves out first or is it your chest that moves first? Your stomach should move out first!

Deep diaphragmatic breathing stimulates the parasympathetic nervous system, which relaxes muscles and allows more oxygen to flow throughout the body. Think of it as calming, rather than constantly breathing into your chest, which is panic breathing and serves to tighten and stress your body. If you need evidence of perfect breathing, then look no further than a baby as they take big full-belly breaths.

To help our clients learn how to breathe right we ask them to practise this drill (as shown in the picture) with a small weight or book on their belly to ensure that, when they take a breath, the weight moves up and down and, most importantly, the breath starts in the belly and moves upwards towards the chest, NOT the other way around. Neck and shoulder tension is exacerbated by excessive and stressful chest breathing.

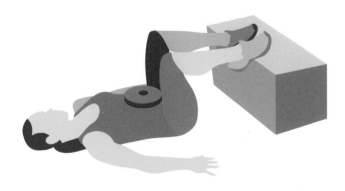

We don't need to make this into a religious experience with a special sequence to follow: simply inhale on a 5-second count, feel your belly pressing out for 3–5 seconds, then exhale on a 5-second count and repeat for 10–20 breaths.

> *If breathing is good then usually movement integrity is good.'*

Perform daily – this is the perfect practice to follow when you're feeling stressed and overwhelmed.

Diaphragmatic breathing also serves as a bracing pattern to help us stay tight in our core when we're going to lift a weight, for example, when deadlifting, squatting and on push-ups. When getting ready to make any lift that requires us to stay tight we need to push air down into our belly and lower back, which will move it out. We then need to tighten our abs and obliques which will lock that air in. This keeps us more stable in our lift and helps to prevent us getting loose and losing form. One of the most common movements we see people not breathing and bracing in is the push-up. Most people think their lack of push-up ability is purely limited to their arms, whereas we most often see it as an inability to brace correctly, which leads to the hips sagging towards the floor.

If you want to get more out of your training and experience some much-needed stress relief, then you absolutely must learn how to develop the power of your breath so you can return to your very nature to breathe right, like you did when you were just a little toddler.

You need to think in terms of at least a six-month cycle to make significant changes to your mobility. Change in this aspect of fitness can be quite slow but it has to be given the time needed to change. That adjustment is not going to be possible if you're constantly erasing your progress from lack of consistency or hitting training sessions too hard and too often with a body that is ill-prepared to handle the workload. In the following chapter we will teach you why progress is progress and having a 'no pain, no gain' attitude isn't necessary to get to your goals.

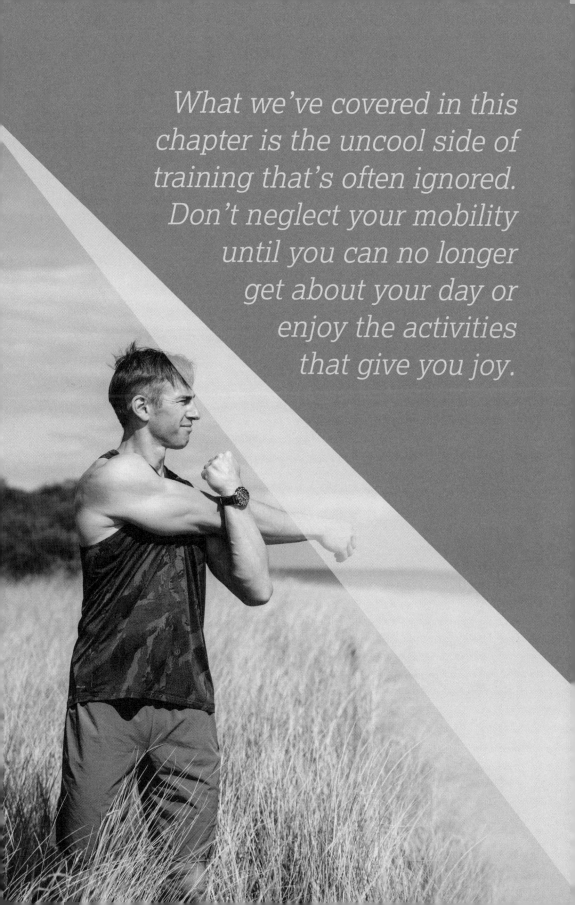

What we've covered in this chapter is the uncool side of training that's often ignored. Don't neglect your mobility until you can no longer get about your day or enjoy the activities that give you joy.

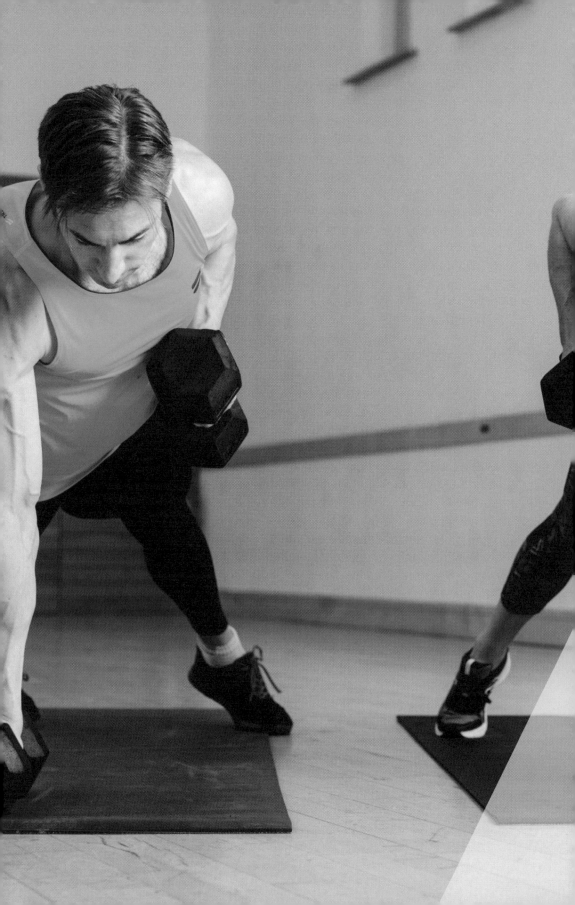

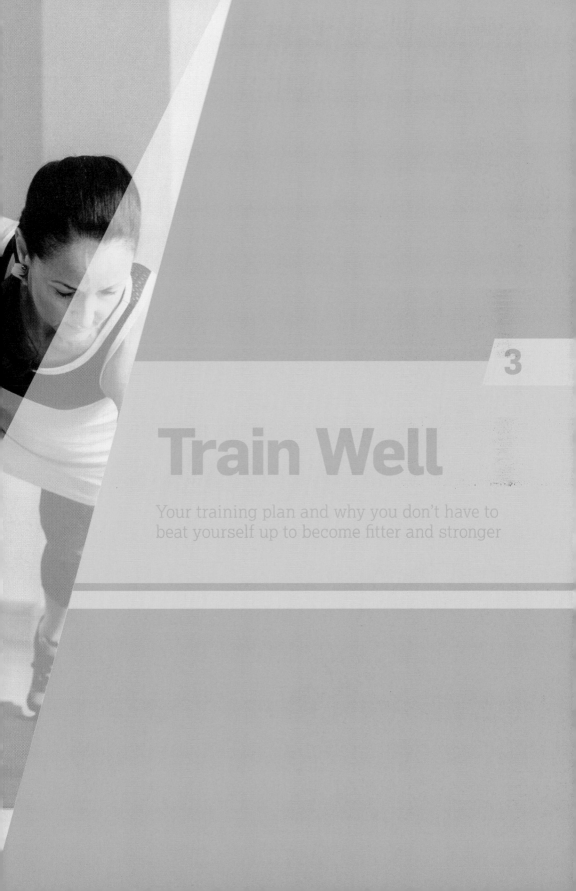

Train Well

Your training plan and why you don't have to
beat yourself up to become fitter and stronger

3

Why sweating doesn't equal progress

We may live in a society where being overweight or obese is becoming the norm but the solution presented to rectify this is often one of 'If it's not hurting then it ain't working'. When I first started working in the fitness industry I had been taught that a 'no pain, no gain' attitude to fitness was the only way to train people. This resulted in unnecessary overtraining as well as injuries and burnout. A 'go hard or go home' approach to training is still common today but it is the wrong approach to a sustainable, enjoyable training plan that will deliver the results you want.

A certain degree of effort and stress must be placed upon the body in order to make progress but when you start turning exercise into a competitive sport then you are going to see problems arise. I firmly believe that where competition starts is where health ends. Professional athletes are often put up on a pedestal as exemplars of physical excellence when, in reality, any interview with a top athlete would tell you they are constantly battling muscle soreness, injuries and fatigue. The mistake of many people is to try to mimic the training and nutrition of the pro whose main objective is high-level performance, yet the average person is looking to get fit and feel his or her best.

In this chapter I want to teach you how to train effectively without exposing you to increased risk of injury, simple ways to measure your overall fitness and why the trend of performing continually high-intensity exercise for most people is harmful and dangerous.

Start assessing, stop guessing

Finishing a workout covered in sweat isn't evidence of progress, progress is evidence of progress. What I mean by this is that we should have certain standards of progress in our training that builds a rounded vision of fitness and to be fit for the life we lead as opposed to falling into the trap of thinking that just because you're making sweat angels on the floor, your fitness is moving in the right direction.

You need to measure three main areas of your fitness:

1. **Mobility**
2. **Strength**
3. **Conditioning**

Mobility

Progress is measured as you become more and more comfortable in the stretches covered. Combine these stretches with any soft-tissue work you need and you will see huge improvements on these tests. I don't mean that you won't be sore from your workouts (you may be). There are plenty of days where I'm stiff or sore from the

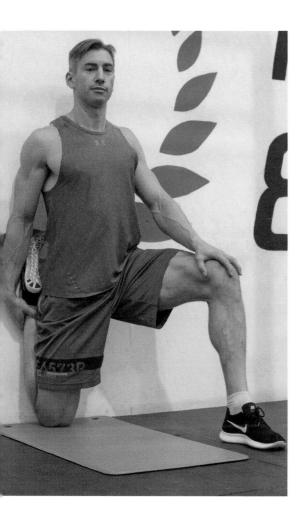

previous day's training and that might push my mobility capacity back a bit, but regaining and returning to normal ranges of motion shouldn't take more than a day or two. There are two main reasons why you will get sore from training:

1. a new activity or movement you've never done before;
2. high training volume or load, i.e. you did more reps or used heavier weights than usual.

Some soreness from workouts is acceptable but it shouldn't be seen as a sign of progress or not.

Strength

The second area to check is your strength. Strength is a vital component to your overall fitness because stronger muscles make any activity easier. There is a point, however, where pushing for ever-increasing strength comes with a cost.

Strength training also increases your base metabolism, which means you can burn more calories while at rest.

All our clients start with the fundamental movement patterns, which are the squat, the deadlift, pressing and pulling. These are not optional movements as we need to have the capacity to move through these ranges of motion for the rest of our lives. We outline how to approach these movements through exercises in the following section.

To show decent upper body strength I recommend that you build your ability to perform a push-up from the floor and a one-arm row (see page 62) using 12–16kg for women and 16–24kg for men or a chin-up/pull-up hanging from a bar.

For lower body strength, a good standard is to be able to do a squat and deadlift or single-leg variation, such as a lunge, step-up or single-leg deadlift with good form

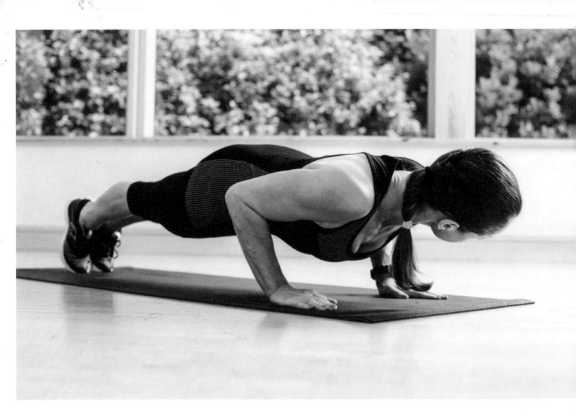

because some of us have lost the range of motion to perform these movements safely. Once this has been established I would like to see everyone build up to using some added load, e.g. on deadlifts, to progress to the point where you can pull your own body weight off the floor.

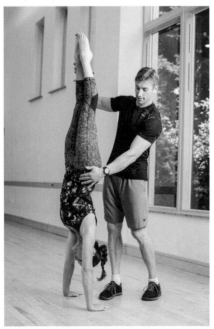

I often see people pushing heavier and bigger weights to get stronger but for many this is unnecessary. There will come a point where strong is strong enough and where fit is fit enough, but I rarely encounter people who are mobile enough to sustain and maintain the fitness and strength they're demanding of their body. Building strength and conditioning can seem more attractive but don't get caught in the trap of working on these elements, disregarding your base mobility and how well you move.

One last element to working on strength is variety. I chop and change the movements I use with clients all the time. You might often read about particular exercises as being better or more effective for fat loss, for example, or muscle tone. Variety is important to a training programme NOT because new or different exercises are radically better but because your body has to adapt to a new training stimulus. As you maintain and show consistency in your training, look for ways in which to vary the movements you use. This can be done through changing how many reps and sets you do, the speed of the repetition, the use of an additional load and how you hold that extra load. Variety is important as long as it's not just variety for its own sake and you are using the change to further your progress on the fundamental movement patterns.

Conditioning

The third area to measure is your capacity to deal with having your heart rate elevated. If you have not been exercising in a long time or you're coming back from a lay-off, the first step is to go for a brisk walk. Walking is one of the most underrated forms of exercises. It is low impact and generally not that stressful to do regularly. Start with being able to walk continuously for 30–60 minutes without getting totally out of breath or excessively stiff the next day. If you have little to no exercise history, then the very last thing you need is a boot-camp or high-intensity exercise class. You

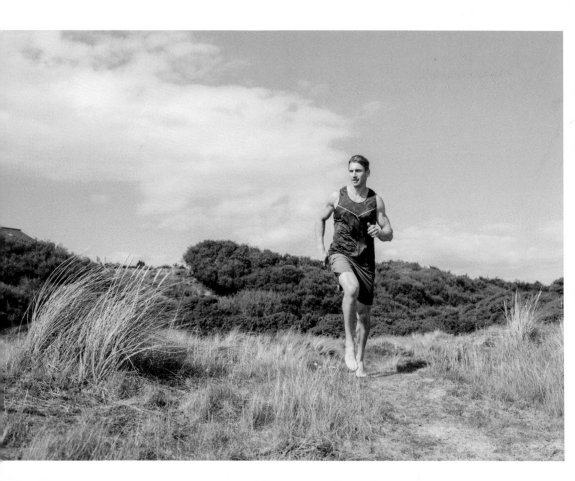

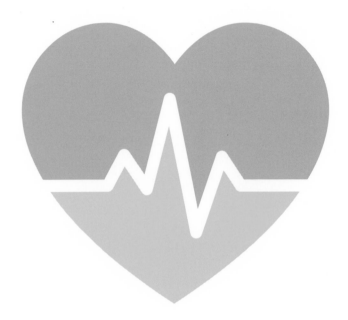

should instead combine regular walking with the mobility and strength work we recommend to build up your conditioning to the point where you can have your heart rate elevated.

As you continue to train with consistency, it's a reasonable goal to be able to do any form of exercise that elevates your heart rate to within 60–70 per cent of your capacity (see facing page) and sustain that for 10–30 minutes. This will develop your aerobic capacity. Building your aerobic capacity first is vital as it allows you to exercise while keeping your heart rate at a manageable level and cope well with the stress exercise places on your body. If your training is not sequenced in this way, what can happen is that every and any form of exercise feels hard and stressful because you have not developed your ability to handle working at a low heart rate first.

Pull back, don't push through

When I was in my early to mid-twenties I trained far too hard and too often and although I looked fit and healthy, I often felt tired and sore. Remember: the goal is to feel and not just look fit.

Our workouts consist of a series of exercises that will both build your aerobic base and improve your strength.

Calculating exercise intensity

There are two options to calculate exercise intensity. The first is a rating of perceived exertion (RPE).[1] Lower rating equals light/easy effort, higher rating equals very intense/max effort.

10	**Maximum Effort Activity** Completely out of breath, hard to keep going, can't talk
9	**Very Hard Activity** Difficult to maintain intensity, barely able to breathe and speak
7–8	**Vigorous Activity** On the verge of becoming difficult to maintain, shorth of breath but can speak a sentence
4–6	**Moderate Activity** Feels like you can exercise for a long duration, short of breath but can maintain a conversation
2–3	**Light Activity** Feels like you could maintain it for hours, easy to breathe and carry on a conversation
1	**Very light activity** Anything other than sitting, sleeping or driving

The second is as a percentage of your maximum predicted heart rate. If you have access to a heart rate monitor, we think it is preferable to use this method as people rarely estimate their perceived effort correctly.

Maximum predicted heart rate = 220 minus your age

For example, Bill is 35 years old. 220 − 35 = 185 beats per minute (bpm).
60–70 per cent of 185bpm = 111–130bpm

I would get Bill to wear a heart rate monitor and keep him within about 110–130bpm as he exercises.

This gives us a starting point to work from and can be adjusted up or down depending on the individual. The mistake I see most often with people new to training is not building up their base first and jumping straight into higher-intensity workouts, which pushes the heart rate far in excess of their aerobic zone and starts tapping into anaerobic exercise. Higher-intensity workouts can be a time-efficient way to train but come with increased risk and are not sustainable as a long-lasting approach to being healthy and fit.

Aerobic versus Anaerobic training

Aerobic	Anaerobic
You produce energy through the use of oxygen	You produce energy without the use of oxygen
Example – exercising at a low to medium and sustainable intensity over a long period of time. Heart rate is in the 60–70 per cent zone	**Example** – exercising at a high to max effort. Performed for short duration in a work/rest interval manner. Heart rate in the >80 per cent zone
Pros	Pros
• Low stress on joints and central nervous system • Increased cardiovascular function • Promotes fat loss • Can be performed frequently if performed for under 30 minutes • Easy to motivate yourself to do something at lower intensity	• Can be completed in a very short time e.g. 4 minutes of work • Can increase cardiovascular function • Promotes fat loss
Cons	Cons
• Needs to be performed for 10–30 minutes When performed excessively can lead to decreased power, speed and strength.	• Can be highly stressful on joints and central nervous system • Isn't suitable for beginners • Can't/shouldn't be done frequently • Hard to motivate yourself to push yourself at really high levels of intensity.

Anaerobic or interval training is often sold to us as being far more time efficient, making you sweat and delivering faster and better results. However, if you're new to exercise then exercise intensity needs to be dialled up gradually or you will experience all the negative consequences of training in that manner.

The same can be said of doing aerobic exercise to excess, e.g. the explosion in those doing marathons, ironman and ultra-endurance races.

Dr James O'Keefe, director of preventative cardiology at the St Luke's Mid America Heart Institute in Kansas city, says:

> When you're sitting around, you heart is pumping about five quarts of blood a minute, and if you run up the stairs hard or push yourself physically, it can go up 35 or 40 quarts a minute … **If you go and run for 26 miles, or do a full-distance triathalon, it completely overtaxes**

the heart. The heart is pumping 25 quarts a minute for hours and hours, and that starts to cause muscle fibres to tear, which leads to a bump in troponin and other enzymes associated with inflammation, and it causes the death of some muscle cells in the heart.[2]

Dr Carl Lavie, medical director of cardiac rehabilitation and prevention at the John Ochsner Heart and Vascular Institute in New Orleans, reported on the ideal dose of running for increasing life expectancy. Among 14,000 runners, the optimal amount of exercise seemed to be about 10 to 15 miles per week. He says, **'Not only did the runners not get more benefit, but the more they did, the faster they ran, the more frequently they ran, the more miles they ran, they actually seemed to lose any benefit to the heart.'[3]**

So where does the balance lie?

I recommend that the majority of your exercise should be a combination of mobility, strength and conditioning. Build an aerobic base first, which usually takes four to six weeks to develop, after which you can introduce some higher-intensity sessions, but make sure harder sessions are programmed no more than once or twice per week.

The great New Zealand athletics coach Arthur Lydiard was a pioneer of distance running and liked weeks of base-building aerobic training. He insisted that 'the last thing you should do is speedwork without the stamina to support it'.[4]

As a rule, when I work with clients I never get them to do their higher-intensity sessions on days where they're feeling run down, tired or stressed as that will just add fuel to the fire.

I rarely recommend the use of sprinting or running for high-intensity intervals because of its associated impact on the joints. Most people don't have the requisite mobility and good running technique to do it safely. When I get clients to do higher-intensity sessions I use low-risk and low-impact movements, e.g. bike, rowing, pushing a sled, or I'll use a combination of exercises they can do with good form with little recovery time so it gives us the same training effect in terms of pushing their heart rate over the 80 per cent range.

Our workouts are designed to enable you to increase or decrease intensity based on how you feel. They are also effective for those who want to improve performance in their sport e.g. golf, tennis, triathlon, cycling and running. Increasing your hours playing or practising your sport will help to a point but this needs to be supported by addressing the two foundational elements of fitness, which are your strength and mobility. The workouts covered will enable you to build strength, conditioning and mobility yet don't expose you to increased wear and tear on your joints.

I have worked with pro golfers who built up to being able to do multiple chin-ups and deadlift well over their own body weight and now play better golf and get injured less frequently. I have also helped triathletes work on their mobility so that their hip and knee pain went away. If you want to play and improve at your chosen sport then you need to work on your weaknesses and address your overall fitness and not just the skill of the sport.

Approaching exercise in this progressive, sensible manner can be difficult to adhere to because you will often try to cure your lack of training consistency with intensity. You feel guilty about eating too much at the weekend so when Monday rocks around you want to cram more effort and intensity into a single session rather than taking the time to build things up. A professional athlete wouldn't approach it that way and neither should you. You need to have most, if not all, lifestyle factors locked down if you want to push your body to its limit, and that means eating well, sleeping well and a job that doesn't have you working all hours of the day and night. A top-level athlete earns the right to push so please don't buy into the dogma of 'no pain, no gain'.

The same applies when you're feeling run down, tired from work or lack of sleep. At times like this, you should not try to 'push through'. Instead, back off the intensity, loading and duration of the session, take more breaks and spend more time on mobility and core work as both are low stress and will set you up perfectly to hit a far better workout the next day.

The goal

It truly is a pity that fitness is often sold to us in sound bites, memes and click-bait headings with misleading articles dished up on social media. I want you to learn that exercise needs to be approached in a systematic way with guidelines of where and what you need to work on so you can look and feel your best throughout your life.

Through training in the manner that I recommend I have been lucky enough to work with some clients weekly and bi-weekly for over fifteen years. This would have been impossible if my training philosophy was 'if it ain't hurting, it ain't working'.

Learn to listen to your body and know on what days to push a bit more and what days to hold back. One of the easiest ways to do this is to take your pulse upon rising in the morning and then average it out over a normal non-stressful work and training week. What you will discover is that days where it is a little higher than normal (3–5 beats per minute higher) will coincide with your training feeling a little harder. If you wear a heart rate monitor you might even see a jump in your numbers in parts of your training that are normally comfortable for you. You won't have as much pep and joints might feel a little achier. Listen to that and dial things down a little.

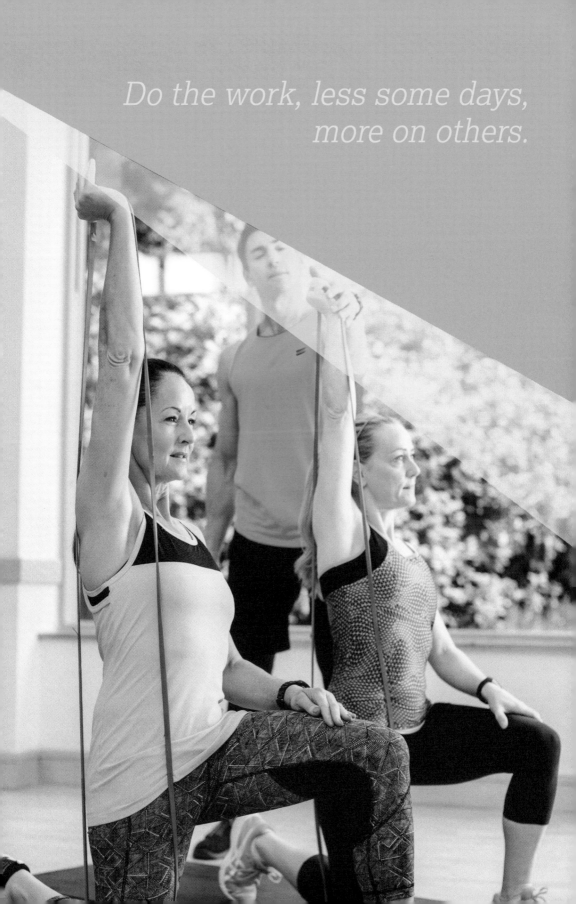

Do the work, less some days,
more on others.

Workouts

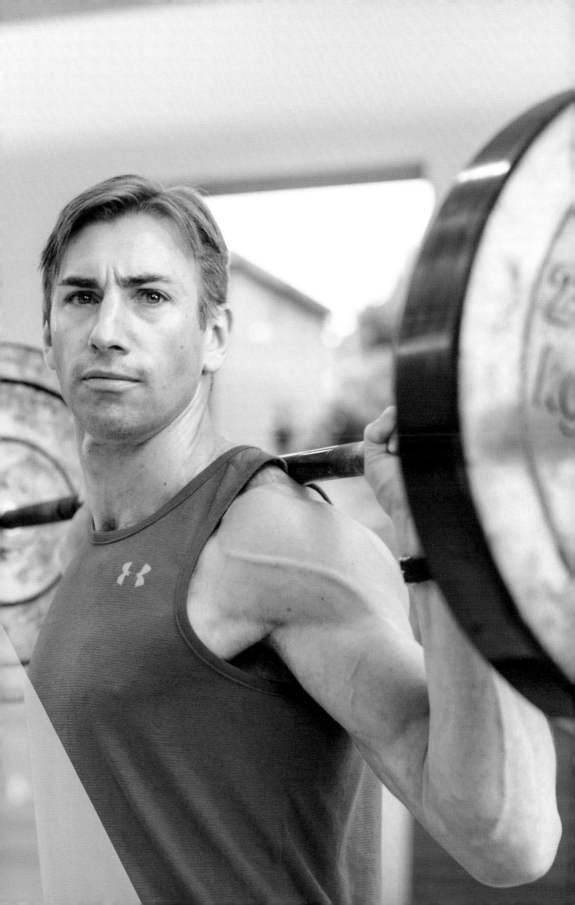

Workouts

The training programme laid out in this section is designed to give you the greatest bang for your buck. You won't need to do cardio separately or attend a yoga class to work on your flexibility. We focus on:

a. The fundamental movement patterns
b. An accessible way to train with limited equipment
c. An integrated approach to addressing all aspects of your fitness – mobility, strength and conditioning

The training is divided into four sessions that are interchangeable – i.e. they don't have to be done in the order listed – and scalable – i.e. they can be adjusted up or down based on your current ability or fitness.

We often get asked: 'How often should I train?' To which we respond: 'Daily.' This might seem excessive so to put this into context what we would like you to do is simply to move daily, e.g. some days this is just going for a walk at lunchtime, followed by some foam rolling and stretching in the evening and the next day use one of the training days provided here. You can then alternate between higher-activity and lower-activity days.

It is not normal to be inactive and spend hours sitting daily. Regular movement helps us maintain all the physiological systems to help lower our risk of cancer, diabetes, heart disease and obesity. Studies continually support the fact that the more inactive and overweight you are, the higher your likelihood of suffering from all forms of degenerative disease.

The main caveat to moving daily is to ensure some element of polarised training. You should have days when you feel good and do much more work and days when life gets in the way and you do a lot less, but the overall result is more exercise in general.

To make changes in your body you need to place it under a certain amount of stress that it is currently not accustomed to. However, if you are coming from a place where you've been very inactive and sedentary for weeks or even years, then daily walking combined with the mobility work provided here might be enough for you to do daily for the first month.

Thereafter, you can pick two of the training days per week and start to integrate them into one week and pick the following two to insert into the next training week. You can stick with this format for weeks or even months. Vary the movements used as your experience expands and over the course of four to six weeks, aim to hit all four workouts in a single week. There are no rules regarding this as you need to listen to how your body feels and do less or more, based on how you feel on a session-by-session basis.

> *Consistency on the basics will always trump how hard you work in a few 'killer' training sessions.*

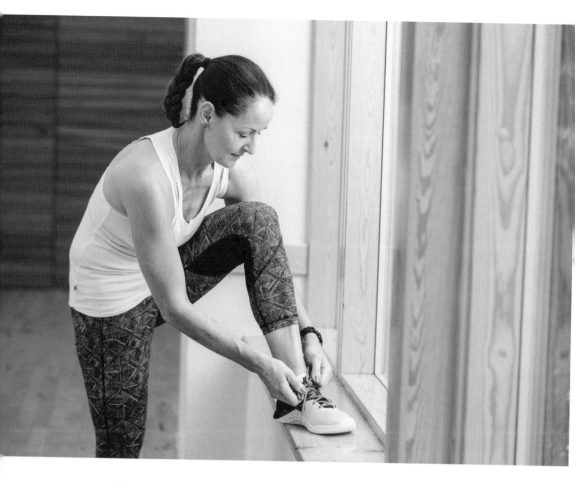

The single biggest mistake we see from those establishing an exercise habit is to overdo it. Your lack of training consistency will never be cured though higher-training intensity.

What we want is a training template that allows you to have the greatest adaptation to the stress that's being placed on your body with the minimum amount of time needed to recover from that stress. Is it really that smart to train so intensively in a single session that it leaves you stiff and sore for days? This leads to a loss of ability to train again or even walk the next day, which goes against our ethos of moving daily. There's no problem in your desire to work hard but many people use hard work as a safety blanket to cover up their inconsistency in eating well, training smart and getting enough sleep. A case in point: notice how busy gyms are on a Monday versus a Friday.

If you've been training regularly then you can scale up the workout templates provided by adding a few more reps or increased load. There is a point where adding more reps becomes redundant and you need to add more load or swap to a more challenging variation of a movement. For example, if you've mastered squatting with your own body weight, you can add load by holding a kettlebell and then play with the tempo of the movement (how fast you move up and down) or insert pauses into the movement, such as holding the bottom of the movement for 3 seconds on all reps.

Your body requires variation in order to keep progressing and these subtle changes help with that process but you must earn the right to variation. It is a waste of time changing your training every week if you are not training consistently.

Why these movements?

We have chosen the movements in our programme because they deliver the quickest and most transferable results to our clients. The training days are a mixture of a lower body movement, upper body movement, a core or midline stability exercise and an exercise that on its own would increase your heart rate. When combined, you have a perfect and balanced mix working on your conditioning as well as touching on strength elements. As clients show progress in their training we separate their workouts into a strength section and a conditioning block where the loading or resistance on the strength increases. However, if you are only starting out training properly in this way then it's likely you will need a mixture of ALL aspects to your fitness, rather than purely strength work OR conditioning work done solely. These workouts can be integrated into a weekly schedule with activities that you currently enjoy, such as yoga or Pilates classes, running, swimming, etc. We have worked with clients who have hugely improved their running or tennis performance by adding just two of our training days into their week. This change gave them the structure to address weak links in their sport or activity, which is often their mobility or base strength.

The programme also covers movement patterns that we need to train frequently, e.g. upper-back pulling exercises to help us draw our shoulders back, deadlifts to help teach us to pick things up off the floor and put them down safely, and squats (because everyone needs a firm butt – right?).

These exercises are what are called the big compound lifts. This means they recruit the largest and most powerful muscles in the body. By activating the larger muscles, this in turn helps us get stronger, and stronger and more mobile muscles make all work easier, ramp up our metabolism and help us look and feel fit and toned. None of this happens to any great extent if your training plan doesn't include the exercises we suggest or if the loading you're using is not significant enough to elicit change in your body.

How hard is too hard?

We suggest that 80 per cent of your training should be done at a low to medium intensity and just 20 per cent is performed to a high or very high intensity. This recommendation stems from polarised training as taken from the Norwegian-based researcher and sports scientist Stephen Seiler. His work has been instrumental to our thinking regarding training intensity as he has consistently shown that the top athletes in the world in a range of sports spend most of their training time at a low to medium intensity. Just one training session in every five is performed at a hard or max intensity.

This is not a new concept and it is a recommendation that one of the most influential running coaches, Dr Phil Maffetone,[5] has been encouraging people to practise for years. Dr Maffetone noticed an increased risk of injury and burnout when athletes were exercising too hard, too often. Through working with hundreds of clients year in, year out, we have observed that many have no issue with wanting to push themselves hard. Our job as coaches is to keep our clients off the physio table and in the gym but we can't do that if they're approaching ALL sessions wanting to work at an eyeballs-out pace.

To counter this we recommend Dr Maffetone's calculator to ensure that when you should be exercising at a low to moderate pace (80 per cent of your training) you have something to aim for.

Dr Maffetone calls it your **Maximum Aerobic Function** (MAF), which is calculated as: 180 minus your age. For a 35-year-old, MAF pace while doing conditioning work should be 145bpm or thereabouts.

Note: you can use a simple heart rate monitor with a chest strap to check these numbers. We've tested monitors that take a pulse from your wrist only and found them to be not as accurate as a chest strap plus watch model.

This number should be adjusted up by 5bpm if you have a strong conditioning base from training, are injury free and generally feel good. It needs to be adjusted down by 5–10bpm if you're constantly tired, recovering from injury, lacking sleep or stressed.

Training at your MAF pace will allow you to train often in a non-stressful manner. It gives you all the cardiovascular, strength and blood-flow benefits of training without the high risks associated with continually training well above this number.

We've worked with many clients who appear fit yet don't feel fit due to training too hard, too often. There's nothing wrong with pushing your heart rate 30–40bpm higher than an MAF pace occasionally but first you need to show the capacity to sustain an MAF pace for 20–30 minutes before you push to those levels. If you train 10–20bpm or higher than your MAF pace all the time, you're living in what **Stephen Seiler calls 'the black hole'.**[6] This level of intensity is not high enough to be truly high yet not low enough to be at an MAF pace.

Black hole training is the absolute worst place to be in your training.

Why is higher not better? You get none of the benefits of the lower work and haven't got the energy to put forwards an honest effort for very high or max effort work; it's the worst of both worlds.

We want you to learn to vary exercise intensity in your training, so on days where you feel good you can push it a bit or a lot more, but understand that you will require more recovery from that session via a day or two training at MAF pace.

Listen to your body

Remember: the goal is to move daily and that is impossible if training makes too much of a demand on you and you don't listen to your body. An easy way to assess your readiness to train is by taking your pulse first thing in the morning. Just swing your legs out of bed, sit upright and take your pulse for 60 seconds. Take an average over the course of a normal week and then notice any jumps in this measurement. For example, if your average pulse per minute was 65bpm and one day after a very stressful day in work or lack of sleep for whatever reason your heart rate is 69bpm, you need to pay attention to that. That's a day to pull back in training, spend more time doing low-stress movement, such as mobility work, walking, etc., and use recovery methods to help get the body back to normal, e.g. foam rolling, Epsom salts bath, sauna, massage, etc.

To ignore this and plough ahead with training and to train at a very high intensity is asking for trouble. You don't need to train with punishment or guilt as motivation. Be kinder to yourself and pull back!

If you want to get slightly more technical you could use a heart rate variability (HRV) app which measures the time interval between heartbeats. Many top sports teams and athletes in the world use HRV apps or monitors to quantify their training readiness. You measure first thing in the morning and the apps typically give you a colour code to how much you should push it that day e.g. green = go for it, red = back off. Over time, you'll become better at getting a feel for it yourself but we've found that most people are terrible at self-assessment initially and don't factor in stress, sleep and other external factors to their training.

The flip side of this recommendation is to be OK about pushing yourself on days when you should work hard. Tough work should be done once per week if your body and mind feel up to it. Avoid judging how your body feels until you get warmed up and moving in your session because you might have a great session once you get the wheels rolling. Listening to your body is not an excuse to do nothing. It should allow you to develop exercise-intensity discipline so that you move often and live in both the lower and higher poles of training zones.

How to apply the training plan

Spend the time needed to read though the instructions for the movements listed and scale up or down according to your ability. At the very least, foam roll and stretch daily, even if it's just for ten minutes. This is even more important if you spend hours every day sitting down hunched over a keyboard.

Some movements might be challenging to begin with but we've found that the more mobile people become, the easier the training. The one big regret we hear time and time again is clients wishing they had spent more time maintaining and improving their strength and mobility.

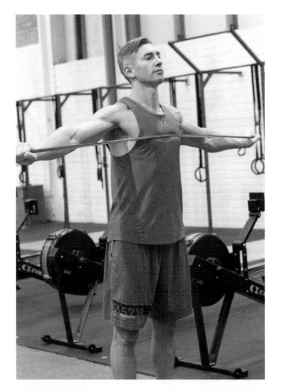

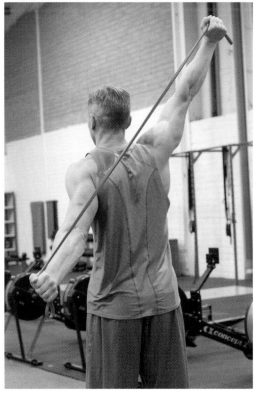

The warm-up

In the warm-up we recommend using bands. We also use them in some strength and stretching exercises we teach.

As an overview, the warm-up is based on the mobility work from the Move Well chapter and would look as follows:

1. Foam roll an area, e.g. thighs. Stretch the thighs using the pigeon stretch. Do some squats holding a post or door frame. Do some forward bends.
2. Foam roll the calves. Stretch them using the single-leg downward dog stretch. Do some squats holding a post or door frame. Do some forward bends.
3. Do the couch stretch.
4. Foam roll the upper back and stretch the shoulders doing the shoulder dislocates.
   Combine these with something to increase your body temperature, for example, one minute of light rowing, jogging, pushing a sled, stationary bike work, skipping, etc., and some band work.

There is no need to spend too long doing this either – about ten minutes is good unless you are severely limited and find the warm-ups difficult. If this is the situation for you then don't move into the workouts and instead spend 20–30 minutes on mobility work, repeat this for three to four weeks and then start to dip your toes in the water with the full workouts.

The workouts

The plan is broken into four sessions a week. If the best you can do is two sessions per week then just pick the first two days (Days 1 and 2) and then on the following week pick out the next two days (Days 3 and 4). Keep rotating through the sessions and be sure to not pick out the same sessions all the time, e.g. don't do only Days 1 and 3 just because you like them best. The workouts are structured in a balanced way to hit different areas and movement patterns on each day.

The purpose of each day is to introduce you to basic movements and get you to work on them. These fundamental movements will elevate your heart rate a little, or maybe a lot if you've not been training in some time. All you need to get started is a kettlebell, dumb-bells if you have them and the bands mentioned in the warm-up and a yoga mat.

You can pick up kettlebells everywhere now and I recommend women pick an 8–12kg one and men a 16–20kg. It depends on your level of prior experience and base strength. If you want to judge it then take one off the shelf and do some one-arm rows with it. If you can do them quite easily then it's too light; if they are very difficult, it will be too heavy.

Each day has three main movements to work on strength and one movement to increase your heart rate. I suggest you do five sets (a set is one round of all four movements). Take breaks whenever you need them. Once you've finished warming up and are about to start the workouts, time how long it takes you to do the session. As you improve, your goal should be to complete the workout in a quicker time. As this improves, try adding load (or more load) to the movements where that applies, e.g. hold a weight as you squat and increase that load in time. If five sets feel like too much for you, then of course do just two to three, stop, do some mobility work and then build it up over time.

Each day should take less than 20 minutes, aside from your warm-up and cool-down, and if you have less time to train then do a quick 5–8-minute warm-up and then perform 10–12 minutes of as many rounds as you can get in on the day you pick to train.

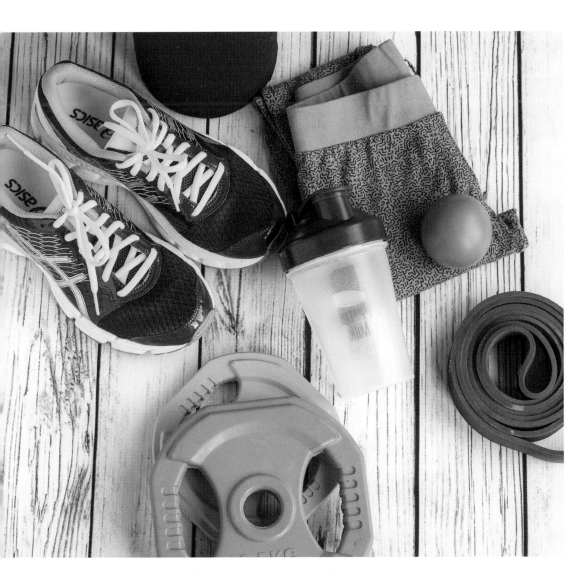

The cool-down

The cool-down should consist of the stretches from your mobility work followed by some soft-tissue work with balls or your foam roller, particularly on any areas which were tight when you started.

Correct form in movements

Remember when you are carrying out the movements, start by making sure that you are standing or kneeling well balanced, and that you mentally prepare before picking up any weight by breathing in correctly and holding your back correctly throughout all the movements.

I show below an example of the correct posture and back position for all movements. You should never overextend your back and, similarly, ensure you are not rounding it.

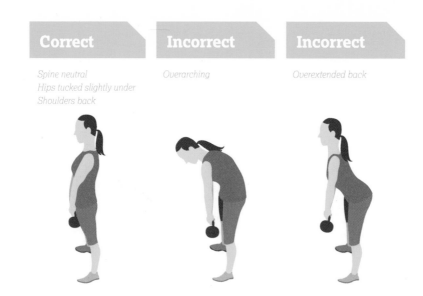

Correct

Spine neutral
Hips tucked slightly under
Shoulders back

Incorrect

Overarching

Incorrect

Overextended back

Common pitfalls when working out

Skipping the warm-up: preparing your muscles for exercise is vital. Work on the areas that have shown up as issues in the Move Well chapter and then foam roll and stretch them daily. If you have just ten minutes to train, spend them working on all the areas you need to get more mobile in so when you have more time to train properly you can feel looser.

Lack of consistency: progress is made one day at a time. Through training and moving daily you will notice improvements relatively quickly but it's long-term consistency that will provide you with the results you seek.

Too hard, too often: if you want to work at higher intensity on any area, let it be on your mobility. Develop discipline around your exercise intensity by varying how much you push in each session.

Strong is strong enough: as you improve you may get to the point where the movements have become easier and you feel stronger and fitter. You might be quite happy to stay at this level so don't feel the pressure to constantly add more or do more as increased load comes with a higher risk of injury. Varying the exercises will keep things interesting and challenging.

Balance: we're aiming for that perfect sweet spot of hitting all aspects of fitness without one dominating at the expense of the others. If you choose to run more and give little to no time for mobility and strength, that will come at the expense of your joints. If you choose to do mainly strength training yet ignore mobility and conditioning work, then expect recovery between sets and sessions to be slower and the risk of injury higher. What's the use of *looking* stronger if you're still feeling unfit when you go up a few flights of stairs?

Your Weekly Workout – Summary Plan

Start a running clock before you begin, to track how long each workout takes to complete. You can aim to improve this time in the coming weeks as you progress.

Day 1	Day 2
Warm-up and Mobility Work 10 minutes	**Warm-up and Mobility Work** 10 minutes
Workout (5 sets)	**Workout** (5 sets)
• Squat 8–10 reps • Kettlebell one-arm rows 8 reps per side • Hollow hold 20–30 seconds • Broad jumps 6–10 reps	• Deadlift 8 reps • Press-up 6–8 reps • Pallof press 6 reps per side with 5-second hold on last rep • Plank tap-outs 10 reps per side and 5–10-second hold in plank after final rep
Stretch and cool down	Stretch and cool down

Progressions to these workouts

There are several ways in which you can make the workouts harder as you progress:

1. Aim to complete the workout in a faster time than you previously completed it.
2. If you started with no weights, you can add weights to the movements, holding dumb-bells or kettlebells, which will make the workout more challenging. If you have heavier weights you can then move to those.
3. You can add more sets.

Day 3

Warm-up and Mobility Work
10 minutes

Workout
(5 sets)

- Reverse lunge 6–8 reps per leg
- Standing or half-kneeling one-arm banded row 8 reps per side
- Russian twists 10 reps per side
- Mountain climbers 10 reps per side

Stretch and cool down

Day 4

Warm-up and Mobility Work
10 minutes

Workout
(5 sets)

- Half-kneeling press 8 reps per arm
- Toes-pointed plank 15–20 seconds
- Reverse curls 10–15 reps
- Kettlebell swings 10–15 reps

Stretch and cool down

Warm-up and
mobility work 10 minutes

Squat

Squat
8–10 reps

Start from a standing position with a shoulder-width stance and toes
pointing out slightly. Sit back and down and make sure you squat so
your hips drop below level of the knees. Drive knees gently outwards.
Keep chest up, butt out and back straight throughout. If you struggle
to do a full squat then hold onto a post or door frame for assistance
to help you get up and down. You could also squat onto a chair/box/
bench that is at slightly below knee height. If your heels keep lifting
when you squat to full depth then stand with just your heels on a

Kettlebell one-arm row

Kettlebell
one-arm rows
8 reps per side

Using a dumb-bell or kettlebell and in a standing position, step
forwards with the right leg. Keep a 90-degree angle in the right knee
and keep left leg straight and with toe pointed outwards, heel on the
floor.
    Place right forearm on the right knee and holding the weight in the
left hand, pull the weight towards the side of the lower chest. Make

Hollow hold

Hollow hold
20–30 seconds

Lie on your back, with knees bent in towards your chest. Straighten
the arms out behind you. Extend the legs and point toes towards the
ceiling. Press the lower part of the back into the floor by contracting
the abdominal muscles hard, tilt pelvis backwards and, as you do so,
lift the chest towards the ceiling so the head and top of shoulders are
off the floor. The arms are still totally straight and almost touching
your ears. Constantly work to straighten the legs as much as you can
so your toes point towards the ceiling. The lower part of the back
MUST remain in contact with the floor as you now start to lower

Broad jumps

Broad jumps
6–10 reps

Mark out a distance of half to full body length on the floor using a
water bottle and towel. Prepare for the jump by standing with feet a
little apart, arms behind and knees slightly bent with chest up. Jump
from one marker to the other, landing firmly on your feet; soften the
landing by hitting a slight squatting position with chest up.
Turn around and repeat. Start with a conservative jump initially

Stretch and
cool down 5–10 minutes

small wedge, e.g. a yoga mat folded a few times, to help with any ankle mobility issues. Perform 8–10 reps on each set. Progression is to move to holding a weight firmly at chest level in your two hands. If you add load, use lower reps, and use higher reps with no load.

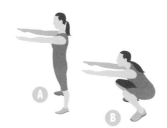

sure the elbow does not drift out as you pull towards your chest. Lower slowly and keep elbow in. Use a heavier load as you get stronger. Repeat on the opposite side.

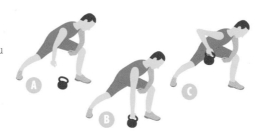

straight legs very slowly towards the floor. The goal is to have the feet about 30 cm off the floor with pointed toes and lower part of the back still on the floor. Hold whatever position has you working strongly to keep the arch out of the lower part of your back as you contract the abdominal muscles hard. Keep your pelvis tilted backwards. Bend knees as much as you need to, to begin with to keep lower back on the floor but work to push legs to straight eventually.

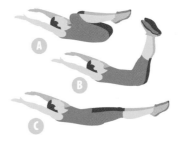

and build distance to body length if possible. Note that over is 1 rep, back is another. You may skip over and back one leg at a time if you need to, at first.

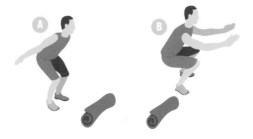

Warm-up and
mobility work

10 minutes

Deadlift

Deadlift
5–8 reps

From a standing position, straddle a dumb-bell or kettlebell in a hip-width stance. Reach down to pick up the weight by pushing your butt back, keeping chest up and a small arch in lower back. Bend your knees about half as much as you would in a squat and think of the movement as a hinge from the waist as opposed to a squat from bending at the knees. As

Press-up

Press-up
6–8 reps

Position yourself facing a firmly rooted table/bench/box that is at about hip height (higher if you struggle with these). Place hands on the table and hold the top of a press-up position, with arms straight, feet pointing forwards, heels off the floor. and tension througout the body. There must be weight placed in your hands so shift your body weight forwards slightly, not back into heels. Lower chest to the table so that your chest – NOT your head – drops between the hands. Press back up. Elbows must

Pallof press

Pallof press
6 reps per side
with 5-second
hold on the last

Loop a band through itself and onto a post, such as in a gym or a banister, anything which is safely and firmly rooted to the ground. Hold the end of the band with both hands clasped together as if praying, fingers interlocked. Standing facing 90 degrees away from where the post is anchored and with hands on your lower chest. Move away from the post so there is some tension on the band, anchor the feet and keep some softness in the knees.

Press the hands from your chest to an arms fully extended position,

Plank tap-outs

Plank tap-outs
10 reps per side
5–10 second
hold in plank
after final rep

Adopt a plank position on a mat and, keeping a tight body line, lift the right leg very slightly off the floor and out to the side as wide as you can without changing your body line. Tap the floor out to the side, return it

Plank hold

Plank hold
5–10 seconds

Start on all fours on the ground. Prop yourself up on your forearms and stretch your legs out with your feet pointed so that you are on the base of your toes and there is a straight line from the shoulders to the heels. Press hard into the legs and hold tension in your abs. Hold for 5–10 seconds and

Stretch and
cool down

5–10 minutes

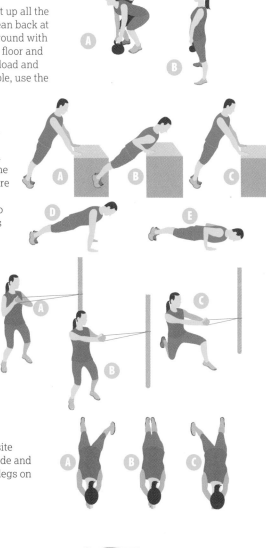

you stand with the weight, keep your chest up all the time, with arms perfectly straight. Don't lean back at the top. Squeeze butt and press into the ground with the legs as you stand. Lower weight to the floor and repeat. As you get stronger, use a heavier load and lower rep ranges; if the weight is managable, use the higher rep range.

move back, NOT outwards, on a press-up. Think of keeping elbows tucked towards your sides but not right against your body. Use lower surfaces as you get stronger. The goal is to perform them from the floor where the chest must touch the floor on all reps. Push-ups can break down quite quickly so don't be afraid to take 5–15-second breaks between reps or after every 2–3 reps.

then return to your chest. Repeat on both sides by turning the other way. On the last rep on each side, pause with arms fully extended for 5 seconds and really feel it in the abdominals. Move further away from the post as you get stronger.

As an alternative, if your post is short then you can do this on one knee with the other leg out in front of you.

back to legs together. Repeat on the opposite side. Start with small movements to the side and increase range as you improve. Alternate legs on each rep.

really work on having tension throughout the entire line of your body. You can work up to holding for longer, up to 20 seconds, as you progress.

Warm-up and
mobility work

10 minutes

Reverse lunge

Reverse lunge
6–8 reps per side

Start from a standing position with feet slightly apart. Step
backwards with right leg and, as you do so, bend the right knee and
gently touch it off the floor. Drive back up using the front leg mainly
and repeat on opposite side. As you get stronger, hold on to weights

Standing or half-kneeling banded one-arm rows

Standing or
half kneeling
banded one-
arm row

8 reps per side

Use a band attached to a post – loop it around itself. Start with the
arm straight and move away from the post so the slack is taken out
of the band and there's some tension on it. Feet should be shoulder-
width apart and facing the post. Pull the hand to the side of the
lower chest. Hand should start and finish in a parallel position
(the same position as you would shake someone's hand). As you

Russian twists

Russian twists
10 reps per
side

Sit on floor with knees bent, arms out in front, holding a light weight
or a book. Recline slightly, keeping back straight and chest up. Go
as far back while keeping tension in the abdomen and your back
straight.
        Twist from side to side, touching the weight or book lightly down
on each side.

Mountain climbers

Mountain
climbers
10 reps per
side

Adopt a press-up position on the floor, hands directly under the
shoulders, body in a perfectly straight line. Don't allow your hips to
rise as you perform the movement.
        Pull right knee to right elbow, return it, then pull left knee to left
elbow. Swap legs on every rep. Keep tension in legs, abs and butt
throughout. Shoulders must remain over the hands throughout.

Stretch and
cool down

5–10 minutes

in each hand or against the chest. Use the lower rep range if you add load and higher reps with no load.

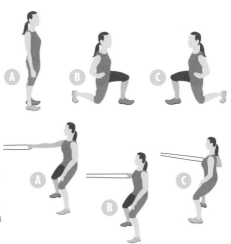

pull to the chest, the chest should move prominently out. Head remains upright and does NOT go forwards. Your upper body should not twist or turn excessively as you perform the movement. Stay tight throughout. As you improve, step further away from the post to create more tension on the band or use a thicker band.

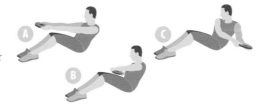

Note that if you round your back when reclining, you have gone too far so sit back up a bit. In the movement, think about making an arc around your body and don't twist as far from side to side if you lose shape.

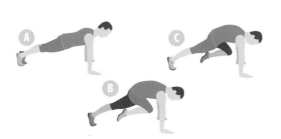

Resist temptation to shift your weight backwards. Keep weight in your hands. Perform the reps in a controlled fashion, not too quickly.

Warm-up and mobility work

10 minutes

Half-kneeling press

Half-kneeling press
8 reps per side

Start by kneeling on the floor. Step one leg out in front so that it is at a 90-degree angle. On the back leg please ensure that the foot is propped up and toes are pushing into the floor. This will give you more support and make it easier to stabilise and squeeze your butt. Using the same arm as the back leg, press a weight or the band from

Toes-pointed plank

Toes-pointed plank
15–20 seconds

Start on all fours on the ground. Prop yourself up on your forearms and stretch your legs out with your feet pointed so that you are on your toes and there is a straight line from the shoulders to the heels. Press hard into the legs and hold tension in your abs. Pelvis should be tucked under and lower back must not be overextrended.

Reverse curls

Reverse curls
10–15 reps

Lying on your back on a mat, pull knees to chest and extend the legs towards the ceiling as much as possible. Place hands on the floor with palms facing down and right next to your bum. Pull the feet back and, as you do so, try to thrust the legs towards the ceiling so that your bum lifts a few centimetres off the floor. You don't need to push

Kettlebell swings

Kettlebell swings
10–15 reps

Use a kettlebell or hold one end of a dumb-bell. From a standing position widen feet to little further than shoulder width apart.
　　Keeping chest up, soften knees, bow from the waist and stand up with the weight.
　　Start by swinging the weight down through your legs then back up to hip or chest height initially. You can start with some mini swings to get a rhythm then gradually swing weight to chest or even

Stretch and cool down

5–10 minutes

shoulder to overhead. The arm should finish right next to the ear and the weight should move up and back, NOT forwards. This exercise can be done with bands as shown and progress to using more weight or a stronger resistance on the band.

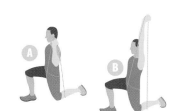

Ideally hold for 15–20 seconds and really work on having tension throughout the entire line of your body. To be sure you are on your toes, think of your toenails being on the floor!

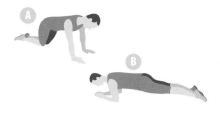

too high. Lower bum to the floor and repeat for 10–15 reps. Keep knees bent as much as you need to at first and, as you get stronger and more mobile, aim to straighten the legs.

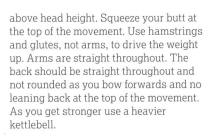

above head height. Squeeze your butt at the top of the movement. Use hamstrings and glutes, not arms, to drive the weight up. Arms are straight throughout. The back should be straight throughout and not rounded as you bow forwards and no leaning back at the top of the movement. As you get stronger use a heavier kettlebell.

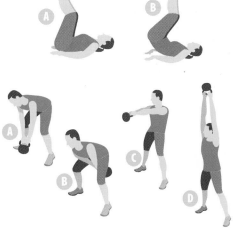

Workout Record Sheet

Keeping a note of your workout, the time you completed it in, weight used (if any), as well as how you were feeling, is great for tracking progress. As you progress by adding weight or increasing the weight you will see your progress here.
(Copy this template to use it as a tracker over multiple weeks.)

Workout Record Sheet: Week

	Day 1	Day 2	
Date			
Time to Complete Workout			
Weight Used			
Notes on how I was feeling			

Workout Record Sheet: Week

	Day 1	Day 2	
Date			
Time to Complete Workout			
Weight Used			
Notes on how I was feeling			

Day 3	Day 4

Day 3	Day 4

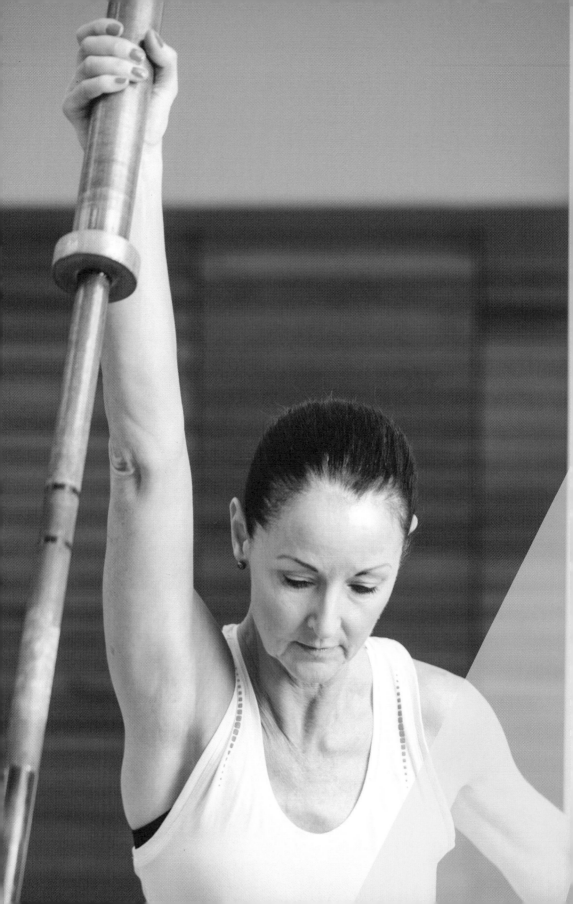

Consistency
trumps intensity

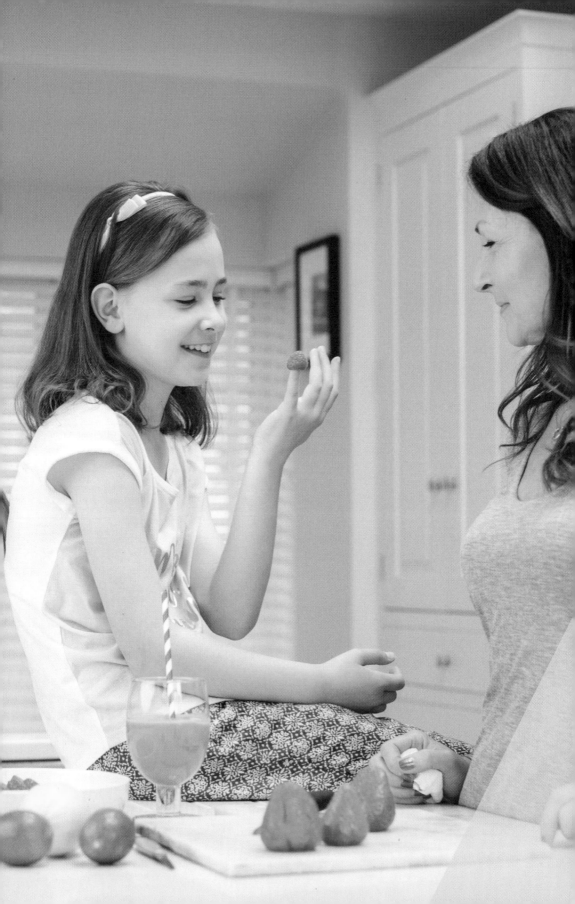

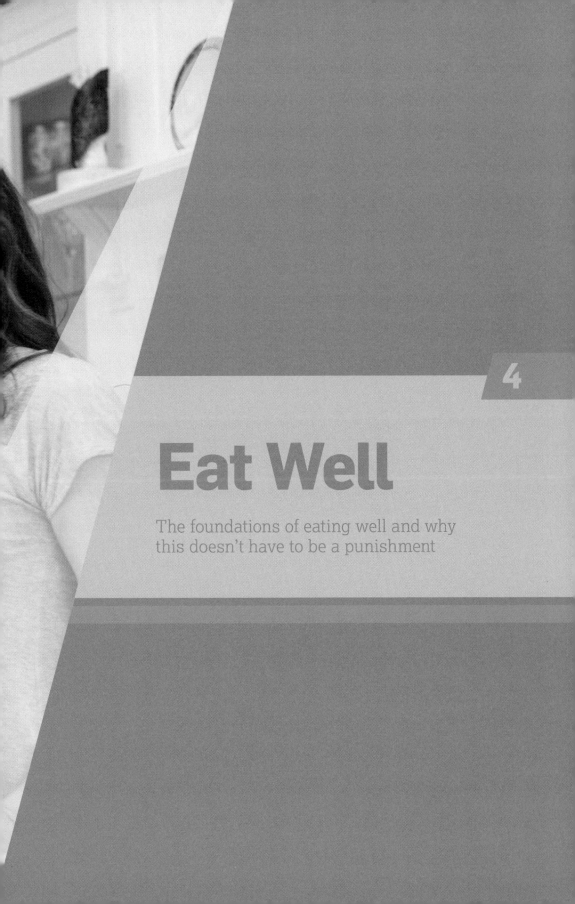

4

Eat Well

The foundations of eating well and why
this doesn't have to be a punishment

Modern life has apparently made food more complicated, with an abundance of food fads, different theories and diets and lots of the latest crazes which promise to deliver a new, fitter, glowing, healthier, lighter you. If it's not gluten-free, it's vegan, vegetarian, paleo or keto.

We like to think we are old school when it comes to our food philosophy, keeping it simple. Food is not something to be conquered; it's not about cheat meals or post-workout protein shakes. '**Eat real food – just not too much**' pretty much sums up our views on what foods we need to give us a balanced, nutritional intake every day. This is not a diet, but a totally sustainable and sensible approach to eating which can apply to everyone.

Nature offers us virtually everything we need in our diet – meat and fish if you eat them, dairy products, vegetables, nuts, plants, grains and seeds – obviously excluding any of those if you have any allergies, such as to wheat, nuts or dairy. We eat practically everything in our house (well, apart from sushi, which none of us likes!) and that includes desserts or baked-goods from time to time. Let's face it: if you are trying to lose weight, these things shouldn't figure too much in your diet because they were probably part of the problem in putting on that weight in the first place. If you don't have weight to lose and have no health problems, then you have more leeway in what you eat. You can afford to enjoy an occasional dessert or sweet treat as long as you feel well on it and the scales aren't going upwards.

In this part of the book we explain the fundamentals of good nutrition, why it's a good idea to track your calories at least for a few weeks if you want to lose weight and how to get started with weight loss, if that is your goal.

We know that if it were as easy as 'eat less and get some exercise', no one would have any problem with their weight and everyone would be really fit, mobile and strong. The reality is that we humans are complex emotional creatures and we eat for all sorts of reasons, far beyond the simple 'being hungry' reason. With this in mind, we look at the importance of behavioural change and getting to the heart of what will motivate you to make a change to eat better, lose weight and feel better. This includes some tips and tricks for getting started, making a plan and coping with temptation when it happens – basically, how to set yourself up for success, how to prepare for nights out to ensure you don't undo all your hard work and how to get the right supports in place so that you can keep going when your motivation might wane. We understand all the common pitfalls, which we have seen over the years working with clients, so you don't have to make them.

If your goal in buying this book was to lose some weight as well as getting fitter and stronger, then it's essential to track your food and count calories, even for a short while. Some people will say there is no need to count calories but to us it is the missing piece of the puzzle if you want to change your weight. The basis of our approach to losing or gaining weight is not just about knowing the value of your food intake but also about bringing conscious awareness to your eating habits. Recording what you eat works because it brings your attention to how you eat, what you eat and why you eat. Understanding your patterns of eating, when you eat well and when you don't, helps you understand your own personal relationship with food. Allying this with getting to know the calorie value of the foods eaten helps you make better choices. It is proven that most of us will underestimate our portion size and calories when asked to take a guess.

To make progress you really have to track and measure!

If you wanted to save money for something important, you would examine your finances, do a budget and figure out how much money you could afford to save every month. The basic principle is the same here: calculate what you need, track and record what you have been taking in, take an honest look at it and make the necessary adjustments. Tracking and recording takes a little bit of time to get used to but we don't ask you to do this for ever – once you get used to meals and portion sizes that work for you, you can drop it. We offer lots of tips and tricks to make this a bit easier and calories are outlined in the delicious recipes that follow, so that the hard work is done for you.

Nutrition principles

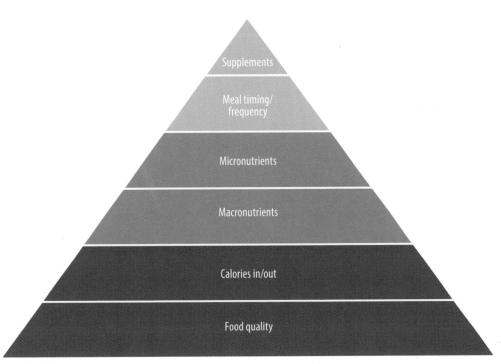

Supplements

Meal timing/ frequency

Micronutrients

Macronutrients

Calories in/out

Food quality

Eric Helms[1]

Food quality

At the heart of our nutrition principles is the belief that we should consume high-quality food. This doesn't mean that you buy only organic food but it does mean that you should buy fresh fruit, vegetables, fish and meat, and cook the vast majority of the food you consume. If you can't cook, do yourself the favour of your life and learn how to, as you will reap the rewards forever. When you can control the quality of what you eat you will feel so much better, as long as you aren't overloading the quantity!

Overall, our bodies require foods that, from a quality perspective, are nutrient dense (contain plenty of vitamins and minerals or, as shown on third layer of the pyramid, your micronutrients), make you feel fuller for longer and are in their natural form, as opposed to nutrient-empty foods (which contain very few vitamins and minerals) that are highly rewarding (make you want to eat more of them) and are processed. An example of that would be eating a dinner with some fish or meat with potatoes and veg versus a small pizza. Both meals may contain the same number of calories but the overall effect on your body is quite different. Eating high-quality foods makes it easier not to have to use so much willpower to keep your nutrition on track.

Calories in/out

While we could debate for a long time the relative position of calories in/out versus macro- and micronutrients on this pyramid, generally speaking, too many calories = weight gain and too few = weight loss.

If you are new to fixing your nutrition and you know your problem is that you consume too many processed foods, start with fixing that in the first month. Ally that with drinking less alcohol and fewer soft drinks and you should see weight loss. You can then move to a more refined approach: calculate your actual calories taken in, map this to your calories required and, from this, work out how to reduce your calorie intake to see further weight loss.

At the heart of these nutrition principles is the importance of understanding the calories you consume and the calories you burn through your daily activity or exercise. Once you develop some insight to this, it will mean that you start to make better food choices. Also, eating real food you have cooked means you will feel fuller for longer and more satisfied.

On page 84 we show you how to calculate your calories required

Calories in/out is the base driver to weight loss, weight maintenance and weight/muscle gain. Many of the clients we work with have a goal of fat loss and the vast majority have been able to lose weight once they have a well-developed motivational plan in place and as long as they have been honest with the calories they were taking in on a daily basis. There are exceptions and for someone who has been obese for a long time, their endocrine, gut health and other systems can be severely compromised, making it much harder for them to lose weight. For many of us, however, this is not the case.

Losing weight is a complicated business. If we were stuck in the jungle with Bear Grylls and had access to just 1,000 calories or fewer per day, virtually EVERYONE would lose weight. However, as we mentioned before, we have enormous access to food and we eat for all sorts of reasons other than just being hungry. Further on in this book we address how to develop your own motivation plan to ensure your success.

The reverse is also true when it comes to muscle gain, i.e. most people who can't put on muscle are simply not eating enough and most need to train harder (especially with weights) in order to generate an appetite that needs filling.

Macronutrients

Nutrients are what we take from the foods available to us and are then used for cellular growth, energy, repair and help drive basic bodily functions. The nutrients we need in large amounts are called macronutrients. They are protein, fats and carbohydrates. Each one provides us with energy in the form of calories and this varies.

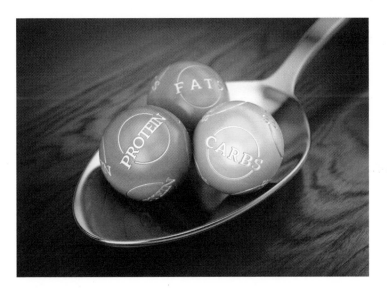

Macronutrient	Calories from 1 gram
Protein	4
Carbohydrate	4
Fat	9

To help you understand this, if a food label states there are 20g carbs, 0g protein, 0g fat, this food will contain 80 calories, all coming from carbs.

Protein

We suggest that you aim to get in roughly 30 per cent of your total energy intake from protein. Protein sources are: eggs, fish, meat and dairy, and there are lower amounts in nuts, seeds, lentils and legumes. We find that most people can hit the 30 per cent recommendation but the quality of the protein you consume needs to come from high-quality sources cooked to preserve the quality. You should aim to consume a wide variety of sources of protein and ensure that it is not all coming from red meat. Don't neglect the plant sources of protein, and eat lots of fish. If you are eating red meat, remember that you will lose some of its benefit if you're regularly taking it in via burgers and a tonne of fries because that process adds more calories, uses vegetable oils which, generally speaking, are bad for us and the quality of the meat is generally poorer in processed commercial beef. If you want a burger, have a home-made one.

We use protein mainly for the production of new tissue and repair of old tissue. It is also a constituent of the enzymes that are vital for digestion and immunity, as well as optimal hormonal production and balance.

Protein is broken down into amino acids and we need 21 of these in various forms. Of this number, nine are essential as we can't make them ourselves. These nine aminos are found in adequate amounts in animal sources but in lower amounts in plant sources. A vegetarian lifestyle can make it a little more challenging to take in adequate protein but it's perfectly manageable if you ensure you are getting in a good balance of amino acids from varying sources.

We don't see a need to increase protein consumption much beyond 30–40 per cent of intake, regardless of your goal i.e. you do not need to drastically increase protein to gain more muscle or drop body fat. Both goals are dependent on calorie intake mainly, not macronutrient intake solely from protein.

One of the great things about protein is that it is a very satiating food which leaves us feeling fuller for longer after meals.

Carbohydrates

We need carbohydrates mainly for energy and generally require them in the largest quantity relative to the other macros. We suggest keeping your carb intake at about 40 per cent of daily calories. This percentage may adjust upwards or downwards according to activity, i.e. if you have a day where you will be doing far more activity or exercise than normal, your overall calorie intake for the day should increase; of that increased intake your carb intake can go up. This shift can move from 40 per cent to 60 per cent of intake.

Carbs are broken down easily and the major organs of the body require adequate amounts to function, e.g. kidneys, heart and muscles. Major sources are vegetables, fruits, bread, rice, cereals, pasta and potatoes.

Another main reason to get in adequate carbs is for fibre intake. Eating processed and sugar-filled foods that contain carbs can limit our fibre intake. Without added fibre, meals become less filling and leave us wanting more.

When choosing your carbohydrates at meal times, aim for slow- or medium-release carbs rather than fast-releasing carbs. However, generally speaking, if you are cooking your meals from scratch you will find that you are eating medium- or slow-releasing carbs most of the time.

Fats

Fats are also known as lipids. Unless you have been medically advised otherwise, we suggest that roughly 20 to 30 per cent of your total energy intake should come from fats. They are a great source of energy but contain more calories per gram – more than double the calories per gram of carbs or protein – so they're needed in smaller quantities.

We need fats for optimal hormone production. They also form the outside cells or membranes that cover our hair, skin and nails, and help the body absorb vitamins.

Fats can be found in nuts, seeds, avocados, dairy, meat, eggs, fish, and coconut and olive oils. Many people still falsely believe that ALL fats are bad for their health and that eating fat makes you fat. This couldn't be further from the truth. It is important to consume fats from a wide variety of sources to provide us with our essential fats, namely omega-3 and omega-6 in the correct ratio. The right balance is as close to 1:1 as possible. This means you should aim to increase your omega-3 fats from oily fish and the likes of chia seeds or linseed; most of us eat too many omega-6s from sunflower oil and other processed vegetable oils.

Excessive fat intake, even of essential fats, can lead to weight gain. This is due to the increased calorie intake: fats are easy to eat in high amounts because of their higher density. This should not make you fat-phobic – the low-fat approach is not the answer for a healthy body, because we need fat for our systems to work effectively. Many of the low-fat products on the market are so high in processed chemicals and sugar that they simply aren't something you should want to put into your mouth.

It is good to understand if you function well on higher or lower amounts of carbohydrate/protein/fats. By function well, we mean feel good and perform well at work and play. You don't have to get too scientific and there is no perfect or ideal breakdown that works for everyone; however, we recommend a split in the order of 40 per cent carbs, 30 per cent protein and 30 per cent fat in the beginning for everyone as it is typically easy to follow and adhere to.

Micronutrients

The easiest way to think about micronutrients is to think of a building with the large bricks being your macronutrients while the mortar is made of the micronutrients, which hold everything together. These are the vitamins and minerals required for everything from muscle growth to cell repair and regeneration. Micros don't act as an energy source and are required in very small quantities.

Vitamins are broken down into fat-soluble (A,D, E and K) and water-soluble (B and C). You need a constant supply of water-soluble vitamins whereas the fat-soluble ones will remain in the body for longer periods of time.

Minerals are calcium, potassium, iron, zinc, etc., and are again required in small quantities. Your body can't manufacture them so they need to be consumed if you want healthy bones, optimal hormone production and a strong immune system.

The easiest way to get in your micronutrients is simply by eating a balanced diet. Some people might ask, 'Can't I just take a vitamin and mineral tablet?' You can most certainly get in your requirements for vitamins and minerals in pill form, but this source may lack fibre and naturally occurring protective substances, such as phytochemicals (important sources of antioxidants which slow down oxidation, a process that leads to cell and tissue damage). We're hardwired to want solid food and will feel fuller after eating real food that requires our body to break it down. It is certainly helpful to take a multivitamin and mineral supplement just to ensure that you cover all the essentials and it can be very helpful if you are training or working very hard but it is not a requirement nor is it a substitute for eating well.

In summary, eat your fruit and veg daily, and plenty of them, because no one ever got fat or unhealthy from eating too much fruit or veg.

Nutrient timing

The nutrition pyramid emphasises that the timing of what you eat is not that important. I believe that nutrient timing only matters when you are doing multiple training sessions per week or even per day. Eating late at night, not having breakfast, etc., doesn't matter. It's what suits you. We are not hung up on everyone (apart from children) having breakfast – lots of people can't eat first thing in the morning.

Supplements

When you eat will NEVE trump how much you eat an the quality of that food.

What supplements do you need? A basic vitamin D supplement in liquid form can help, especially in winter in Ireland when sunlight, which provides it, can be scarce. An all-round multivitamin can be helpful just to cover all bases. Some people can really struggle to get in enough protein so we recommend a whey protein powder, which can be added to smoothies in the morning or simply taken diluted with your milk of choice. Take it once or twice a day.

We are also fans of fish oils, digestive enzymes, probiotics and glutamine daily but that's really dependent upon how you feel and how much you train. Generally, if you're training five to seven days a week your needs can increase and getting vital nutrients only from food can be a bit more difficult unless you are very well prepared.

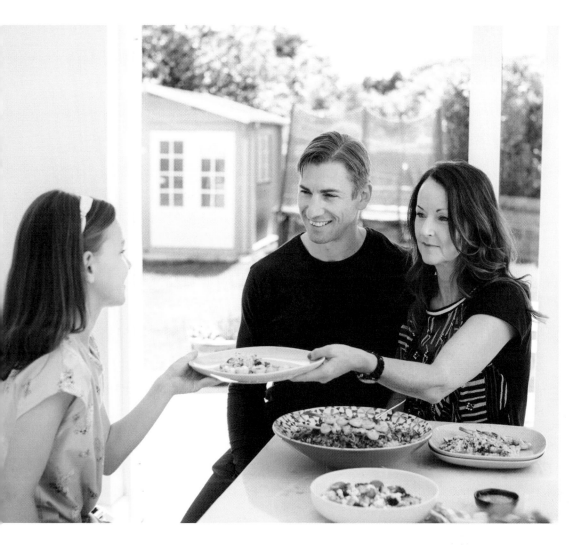

How many calories do I need and how to do the maths

All models are wrong but some are useful.[2]

While it is impossible to be exact in terms of your unique calorie requirement, you can get a pretty good indicator using one of the calorie models available. Calculating calories matters because it is one of the missing pieces of the puzzle in losing weight. Saying 'eat more healthily and do a bit more exercise' isn't targeted enough if you want to lose weight. We recommend knowing how many calories you need and how many you take in in order to achieve your weight-loss goals. We like to use the Mifflin St Jeor calculator.[3]

This will give you your basal metabolic rate or BMR, how many calories you need daily just to get by with zero activity. Once you have that number, you calibrate it according to your level of activity.

Below is an example on how to calculate it. Note that it is different for men and women.

Men

(10 x weight (kg)) + (6.25 x height (cm)) – (5 x age (y)) + 5

e.g. If Tom is a **30**-year-old, **180**cm, **80kg** man this would work out as follows:

    (10 x **80**) + (6.25 x **180**) – (5 x **30**) + 5
    (800) + (1,125) – (150) + 5 = 1,780

This is Tom's basal metabolic rate.
Tom trains four times per week (moderate exerciser) so we multiply by 1.55 to calculate maintenance calories. (See activity multiplier table on facing page). This gives us 2,759 daily calories for Tom to remain at his current weight given his activity level.

Women

(10 x weight (kg)) + (6.25 x height (cm)) – (5 x age (y)) – 161

If Jane is **25** years old, **156**cm tall and weighs **60kg**, this works out as follows:

    (10 x **60**) + (6.25 x **156**) – (5 x **25**) – 161
    600 + 975 – 125 – 161 = 1,289

This is Jane's basal metabolic rate.
Jane trains three times per week (light exerciser) so we multiply her BMR by the activity multiplier 1.375, which gives us 1,760kcal daily. These are maintenance calories to maintain current weight.

Activity multiplier table

Sedentary (little to no activity)	1.2
Light exercise (sports/trains to 3 times per week)	1.375
Moderate exercise (sports or trains 4–5 times a week)	1.55
Active (e.g. an active job and exercises 5–7 times per week)	1.725
Highly active (very hard physical job and exercises every day)	1.9

See page 87 for a handy template to work out your numbers.

Spend two weeks tracking and recording your calories honestly and then you will have your actual daily intake. If you have weight to lose, the chances are this actual number is higher than your ideal maintenance calorie number. You may notice that you are quite good during the week but go off the rails at the weekend. This is common enough and noticing this pattern will be really helpful for you in identifying some of your barriers or challenges to losing weight, which you can prepare for.

Reducing calories

If your goal is weight loss, you need to reduce calories. This should not be a drastic amount: start with a 10 per cent reduction and combine with regular exercise. You will soon see results. As you get stronger and fitter, your muscles will burn more calories than at present so the benefits of your exercise, apart from making you feel better and happier, are even more!

If your actual calorie consumption is considerably more than your ideal maintenance calories, we advise gradually moving to the maintenance figure by reducing your actual figure by 10 per cent every two weeks or so until you reach your maintenance level. This should show results. We recommend you stay at this figure for a number of weeks in order for your body to get used to it. Keep on track using the motivation techniques we have included (see page 94) and don't allow yourself to slip back to the higher figure.

If fat loss is the goal and the scales are still not shifting down, then you may need to lower your calories a little more. Do so, but not so much that you feel miserable and constantly tired and hungry. This won't be sustainable and will make it much harder for you to achieve your goals.

Calculating the macronutrient breakdown for your daily calories

So now you know what your daily calories are going to be. The next step is to check you are getting these from all the **macronutrients** your body needs.

You can use a macro calculator online and punch your numbers in.

If we return to our example with Tom, who hasn't been as active as he said and now wants to drop some body fat, his numbers based on a 40/30/30 split would look like this:

Total maintenance calories per day: 2,759
Drop by 10 per cent, i.e. reduce by 275: 2,484

Breakdown	Carbs 40%	Fat 30%	Protein 30%
Total calories 2,484	993	745	745
Grams	993/4 = 248g	745/9 = 83g	745/4 = 186g

Once you have worked out your numbers, you can track your food intake using the recipes we have suggested. If you are eating other foods use a handy app, such as My Fitness Pal, to make this process easier.

This might sound complicated and it will need minor adjusting because your numbers may need to go higher or lower depending on your progress or lack of progress. However, it takes the guesswork out of the process and once you have a base number to begin with you can use a diary or a calorie-tracking app to check how close or far away you are from your goal calorie numbers on a daily basis.

The alternative to all of this is to guess how many calories you're taking in most days, which can work fine in the beginning if you are moving from a place where your nutrition was filled with processed foods and drinks, but in time you will need to go through this process if only to see where you are going wrong/right.

It would be helpful for you to do monthly or bimonthly body fat tests to assess your progress. If this is not possible, taking start and progress photos for your own use can be helpful. They will also help keep you going as you can look at the starting pics and see how much improvement there has been since you began – there is nothing like some positive results to keep you motivated.

If you are groaning at the thought of this, we understand. It might seem like a bit of hard work but the reality is that you need to know what you are consuming so that you can reach your goals. You can also make this easier by introducing predictability into some of your meals.

Most of us have a pattern and predictability in what we eat – and if you don't, we suggest you get one as it makes it easier to know your intake. Have a number of similar meals during the week that have a good nutritional profile and for which you already know the calories and macronutrients – this is really handy to know.

For breakfast I will always have a flapjack or yoghurt, plus a piece of fruit, or I'll have a poached egg and some wholemeal toast – having similar meals help you track easily.

Do people at their right weight do this?

The answer is mostly no, because they already eat well, they know the portions that work for them, their diet is pretty good most of the time and they are active with some form of exercise. They have more leeway because they are already in good shape.

But you can get to this position too. When you have lost weight, when you are feeling much better, feeling fitter, sleeping better, feeling happier, when you know what food works for you and what represents good portion size, you can drop the tracking and know that it is OK to have dessert from time to time.

Template

Male 0 x weight (kg) + 6.25 x height (cm) – 5 x age (y) + 5		Female 10 x weight (kg) + 6.25 x height (cm) – 5 x age (y) – 161	
(1) Weight in kg:	x 10 =	(1) Weight in kg:	x 10 =
(2) Height in cm:	x 6.25 =	(2) Height in cm:	x 6.25 =
(3) Subtotal (add 1 + 2)		(3) Subtotal (add 1 = 2)	
(4) Age:	x 5 =	(4) Age:	x 5 =
(5) Subtotal (subtract line 4 from line 3)	=	(5) Subtotal (subtract line 4 from line 3)	=
(6) Add 5 This is your BMR before activity level is added		(6) Subtract 161 This is your BMR before activity level is added	
(7) Activity multiplier (see page 84) (Be honest!)		(7) Activity multiplier (see page 84) (Be honest!)	
(8) Total from (6) multiplied by the activity multiplier in (7). This is your total mainentence calorie requirement		(8) Total from (6) multiplied by the activity multiplier in (7). This is your total mainentence calorie requirement	
(9) Tracked actual daily calories		(9) Tracked actual daily calories	
If I have a weight-loss goal, subtract 10 per cent Goal daily calories		If I have a weight-loss goal, subtract 10 per cent Goal daily calories	
If I have a muscle- and weight-gain goal, add 10 per cent Goal daily calories		If I have a muscle- and weight-gain goal, add 10 per cent Goal daily calories	

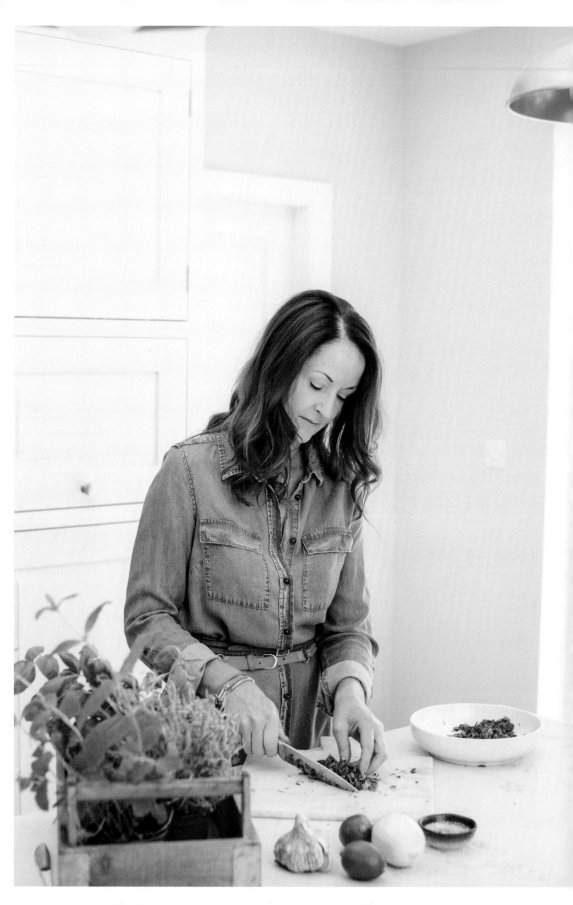

Getting started with eating well

Cooking skills

Cooking is one of the greatest skills to equip yourself with to enable weight loss. Cooking your own food ensures you know the quality of what has gone into it and that it isn't loaded with hidden sugars, fats, additives or preservatives. I personally think there is a great amount of pleasure to be had from making something yourself that tastes good and that you can enjoy with a partner or the family. If you can't cook, make a resolution to learn a small number of dishes that you would enjoy being able to prepare. You don't even have to be able to afford a cookery course, as there are loads of free resources online to show you how to prepare some easy, tasty dishes.

Portion control

I strongly believe in the need for portion size to be related to how active you are and your size. I always ensure that the kids' portions are kids' portions and, generally speaking, females tend to be smaller and have less muscle than males and so their portions should be smaller. My portion is never the same size as Dominic's. I'm smaller than Dominic and don't work out the amount he does. I am quite active, with a good bit of muscle, but there is no way I need the same amount of food as he does. I apply the same principle when eating out and, even though we get the exact same portion size, I rarely eat it all. I'm not being sexist: it's about eating for your size and requirements, so if you are female then, in general, you don't need to eat the same portion size as your brother, partner, male friend, etc. If I'm not sure about portion size, I eyeball it relative to my hand, i.e. a protein portion the size of my cupped palm, two cupped palms of veg, one of rice, potatoes or pasta.

A word on bread

I don't think I would be alone in saying that I love bread and, for me, memories are made of bread because it was the first thing I was taught to bake by my mum. It is, however, one of those foods where portion control is key, especially if, like me, you load it with butter too. If you can and do eat bread, we favour the artisan bread approach where the bread is made using age-old techniques, giving it appropriate time to rise. We particularly love sourdoughs, especially those enriched with seeds and nuts. Better still, if you like to bake then try your hand at making it at home. The same goes for people who suffer from coeliac disease or gluten intolerances: there are lots of gluten-free flours available if you would like to try and bake your own. Just remember to go easy and don't eat it all at once!

Alcohol

We believe that a small amount of alcohol in your diet is fine and has health benefits, not just from the drink itself but also from the enjoyment you get sitting round a table chatting with friends or in front of the fire on a cold winter's evening, taking the time to hear how your other half's day went. The problem is that for many of us, it isn't the odd drink but a half bottle of wine a few nights a week and much more at the weekend. Excess alcohol has no role to play in being healthy and fit.

First, consider the calories in most drinks. Many of us don't even think about this when having a drink. Secondly, think about alcohol's impact on our willpower and motivation – how many of us have hit the crisps or the chipper after a few drinks? This is aside from the negative impact alcohol has on our body – on our liver, heart and brain, and on our sleep. I am not talking about those of us unfortunate enough to suffer from alcoholism and the adverse health and social impacts this has; I'm simply talking about when we overdo it at the weekend or on a night out. Too many drinks and you wake up dehydrated, with a headache and perhaps a queasy stomach; you have to lie on in bed to recover, so any plans for that day just went out the window. Then you usually get a downer, which is actually your brain compensating for any euphoric high experienced the previous night while having the few drinks – you aren't imagining it: the fear and depression post too many drinks is real. So, drink responsibly, know your limits and don't drink your weekly allowance in one day.

The big fat debate

There is no question but that fried processed food contains fats that are bad for you. However, it is important to remember that not all fats are created equally. Good fats are essential for the body and need to be included in our diet. Remember that you get double the calories per gram of fats than per gram of protein or carbs, so be mindful when preparing foods, eating coconut, avocados or putting dressings on your salads. You can still fail to lose weight, even when eating these healthy fats.

Your environment

There are loads of studies which show how your environment impacts on your willpower and that simply having food on show in your kitchen can result in consuming excess calories because it is visible. It is also shown to be less stressful when there isn't a load of stuff crowding countertops and spilling out of bowls, tempting you everywhere you look. Put temptation out of sight as it is easier to control your environment than your willpower.

Shopping

Whether you shop online or in person, do the weekly shop only when you have planned what you are going to eat for the week. Decide what meals you will have, figure out if you're having friends over for food and therefore what extra stuff might be needed, and then do the shopping. Never shop without a list of meals for the week. There are loads of benefits to this – you are not spending extra on stuff you don't need, you'll waste less food as you won't have bought too much that will end up getting spoiled and dumped in the bin.

Try not to impulse-buy so you should also never shop when you are hungry! Sometimes I do go off-piste if I see some lovely piece of meat or fish I haven't cooked in a while or a new recipe catches my eye, but usually I shop by deciding what the week's menu will be, making a list and sticking to it. If you have mentally prepared for the week, thinking about what you will cook and the food is in the house, then you are less likely to call for takeaway.

Make things easier for yourself – don't buy it!

Loading the cupboards with chocolates, sweets, fizzy drinks and crisps just makes things really hard for you if you are trying to lose weight and, really, we all know they shouldn't be there anyway. They are all full of empty calories and are addictive to many of us, and as for fizzy drinks – they are just a delivery system to get sugar and other rubbish straight into the bloodstream.

If there is an expectation for these things to be available at home then you should enlist the help of your household in your plan to get fit and lose weight. Explain that you don't want to have them in the house any more so that you won't be tempted. They should (albeit maybe reluctantly) understand and agree with your plan. If you have a house full of kids who are used to having these kinds of treats available, even for occasional consumption, then perhaps do as we do and just allow the single bar of chocolate or small pack of jellies to be bought on the day that you agree they can have them. I know I couldn't possibly tell my daughter, Eva, that she can't have chocolate or jellies ever again, nor would I want to. I remember the joy of getting sweets when I was a child. However, it shouldn't be a daily occurrence. They aren't in the house but they are bought for Eva at the weekend or on a special day out. The exception to that is fizzy drinks, which are a very rare occurrence in our house. None of us has ever developed a taste for them so apart from times like Christmas, or summer holidays abroad, we just don't have them.

Nutrition

Typical values
(cooked as per instructions)

	per 100g	per 1/4 pack	% adult GDA 1/4 pack	GDA children (5-10 yrs)
Energy kJ	1007	2014		
Energy kcal	241	482	24.1%	1800
Protein	8.4g	16.8g	37.3%	24g
Carbohydrate	20.6g	41.2g	17.9%	220g
of which sugars	1.8g	3.6g	4.0%	85g
of which starch	18.8g	37.6g		-
Fat	13.7g	27.4g		-
of which saturates	5.7g	11.4g	39.1%	70g
mono-unsaturates	5.9g	11.8g	57.0%	20g
polyunsaturates	1.5g	3.0g	-	-
Fibre	0.9g	1.8g		
Salt	0.50g	1.00g	7.5%	
of which sodium	0.20g	0.40g	16.7%	

GDAs = Adult Guideline Daily Amounts are bas...
female. GDAs are guidelines and personal rec...
...ending on age, gender, weight and acti...

Learn to read a food label

This is a really useful tool in our arsenal. I always look at recommended portion size first and the number of calories in that. Check if the portion size seems reasonable or would you have to eat two portions and hence double the calories?

Check the ingredient lists for things you actually know and understand. If there are lots of words ending with '-ose' and '-ase', these are probably sugar so check the carbohydrates and the 'of which sugars' gram amount. As a rough guide, approximately 4 grams is a teaspoonful.

Look at the protein portion. You can calculate the calories from this by multiplying the grams by four. If I am caught on the go needing to buy prepacked foods I always look for a decent protein source as it will make me feel fuller for longer.

Finally, check the fat grams and remember that 1g of fat is 9 calories. Even healthy foods like nuts, coconut, and avocados will contain high amounts of calories because of this.

Make your wellness plan and run it like a project – 'Project Me'

I spent most of my working life on project work and while the projects were hugely varied they all had many common characteristics, the first being that an organisation had decided a particular problem was sufficiently important that attention needed to be focused on it in order to solve it. Over the years I have learned why projects succeed or fail and I have loads to scars and war stories about when things went well or not, but it struck me that the best approaches and learning from this work could be used in the same manner to help people to make change in their life – why not think of it like a project that needs really good planning, goal setting and actions with timelines, contingency plans and regular progress reports? I mean this in a good way – why not devote the same level of attention and detail to yourself as you would if you were doing something important at work or for your loved ones? Wouldn't that attention and focus help you on your project to get fit and lose weight?

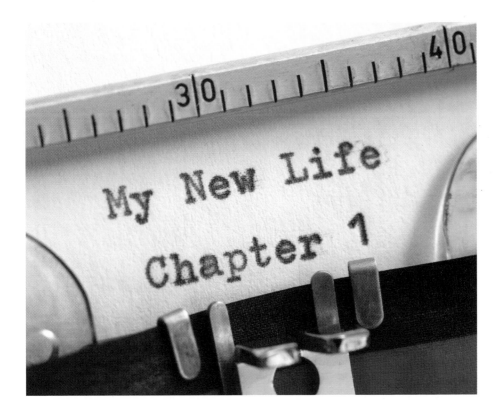

Finding your motivation

If getting fit is a first for you and you also want to lose weight, it will be really helpful for you to spend some focused time thinking what making these changes will mean for you, how your life will be so much better when you are able to move better, are stronger and are the weight you would like to be. How much better you will feel! How pleased with yourself and your achievements you will be! Figuring out your motivation will really help you stay on track when it gets tough and when you want to skip that workout or break out the sweet stuff. It is helpful to develop an image of what you are aiming for – imagine it, write it, draw it, whatever works for you, and stick it on the fridge or somewhere you can see it. If you think you would do better working with someone who can help you with this, look for the services of a health and wellness coach who can act as your ally in undertaking this get-fit-and-lose-weight journey. When you are developing this vision, pick something realistic. Today's supermodel types with six-packs are the result of good genetics combined with working out every day and watching everything they eat. It might look good on Instagram but it's not real life, so develop a vision around what is important to you and right for you, is realistic and enjoyable. For me, I love to work out because I love how it makes me feel and I love feeling strong, but I also work out because I want to stay as healthy as I can for my beautiful daughter. I want to see her walk down the aisle (if that's what she wants) and I want to be able to play with my grandchildren, (again, if she chooses to have them).

Decide

When I say decide, I mean *really* decide – in the pit of your belly decide that you want to do something about getting fitter and losing weight. This isn't a vague 'I really should get fit' where nothing happens or an 'I must lose some weight' thought which flits in and out of your consciousness, but an actual firm decision that you are going to do this. It's amazing how forcing yourself to say it out loud will show you how ready you are to make the change. If you say this out loud, listen also to your gut: it will tell you if you really mean it. Be honest. If you don't feel like you really mean it then it means you aren't ready **YET** to make those changes. Don't give up, though: read this book, figure out what making these changes will mean to you and keep working at it until you can shout out loud that you are ready and able to make the changes needed to achieve your vision.

Learn from past experiences

If you have tried and failed before to get fit or lose weight then spend some time thinking about what happened. You can feel beaten down if you have failed before but try to reframe that in terms of using it as a learning experience for this time. Don't make your goals too hard and unrealistic. There is no point telling yourself you are going to work out six days a week if you know that is not a realistic goal with work, life and family responsibilities.

Be SMART with your goals

Start with goals which are clearly defined for you and are a bit of a stretch but not so unlikely that you won't be able to attend to them.

Specific
Measurable
Attainable
Realistic
Timely

An example of a SMART goal is 'I will walk to work three days a week, on Mondays, Wednesdays and Fridays, and I will do my workout three times per week on those evenings for 30 minutes each session'.

Once you have made your objective, get it into your schedule: write it on your calendar, put it in the diary. If you have family, make sure they can see it too. This activity of recording will raise your awareness and make it harder to skip – it makes you more accountable to yourself, which will help you stick to your goal.

Understand your motivation

Understand how you are motivated – do you like alone time and if so, perhaps that is the time to stick the music on and get the walk/run/workout done. Is there a sport you loved and you would love to get back to? Now is the time to pursue a previous passion.

Enlist support

Do you need people around you to get motivated? If so, get some friends involved in your health and wellness pursuit. Get everyone to set their own goals and get working out together. If you have family, share with them your plans and aspirations – ask for their support and, better still, get them involved. If you have young kids, get out walking together. Some of the best chats I have ever had with my daughter have been during a walk when it was just the two of us.

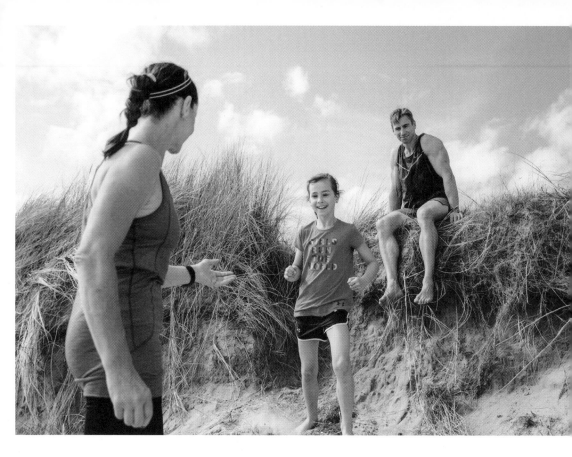

Make contingency plans

We all know that life can get in the way, work can get very busy, family can need you unexpectedly so it will help to think about these in advance and decide how you will handle these challenges if they arise.

Write down what might happen and how you will plan for it so that it doesn't take you by surprise and you don't fall back into old habits of poor eating or no exercising.

When you are really busy at work

If work gets crazy and it seems like you won't be able to do as much exercise, rather than cutting out your workouts altogether you should plan to stick to the schedule but reduce the time spent. This is prioritising yourself, and exercise will help you perform at work. Ensure you are organised to bring your meals into work so that you will be able to stick to your healthy-eating choices. Don't be afraid to tell your colleagues at work – ask for their support either to keep the cakes away or to join you on your journey. Remind yourself that no matter how busy you get, you will perform better if you nourish your body well and take some exercise. If work becomes insanely busy or there are significant other issues to deal with, don't add stress by trying to do too much at any one time. Focus on cleaning up your diet as much as possibly by taking in lots of fresh fruit, vegetables, fish and meat, and get good sleep.

Sleep quality is really important – get a good sleep routine, get electronic devices out of the bedroom so you switch off properly and get up ten minutes earlier than normal to set your intentions for the day and get your lunch prepared.

Special occasions

It's a good idea to plan in advance for special occasions, such as weddings or weekends away. Prepare in advance by checking out the menu and deciding what you will eat and drink, and work out how to make the best decision in a challenging situation. Don't starve yourself all day. That will only be counterproductive as you are likely to go completely off the rails and overeat or, worse still, a drink will go completely to your head. If it is a dinner out, make good choices and perhaps choose just two courses rather than three. If it is drinks and a buffet, fill your plate with your selected food and when you have eaten, leave it at that. There are loads of studies that show if you just graze and nibble, you will eat far more than you realise and than if it was all loaded on the plate in front of you.

If you get sick

If you get sick and are poorly enough to be in bed then obviously, no training until you are feeling better. If you still have an appetite, now is the time to feed your body with healing, nourishing foods. Have soups or food with lots of fresh ingredients. Don't worry if you aren't hungry for a while: just go with whatever your body is telling you and when you are on the road to recovery, ease back gently into the workouts.

Cold Remedy Drink with Lemon, Lime and Ginger

I love this and have been making it for years. Whenever I sense a dose coming on, it really helps. Our daughter has taken to asking for it in the evening before bed – I think she finds the warmth comforting.

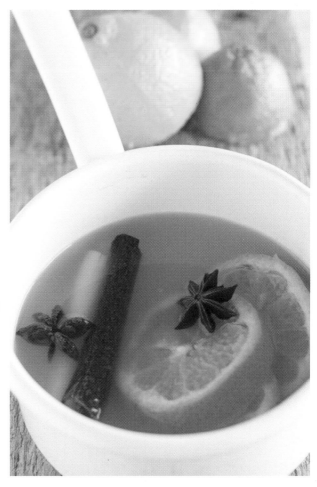

Serves two
2–3 cm piece of fresh ginger, peeled and grated
1 stick of cinnamon
Juice and zest of 1 lemon and 1 lime
1 tbsp honey
1 star anise
Some orange peel, if you have it

Add everything to a heatproof container (or a teapot). Cover with two mugfuls of boiling water and stir. Leave to infuse until cool enough to drink. Strain and enjoy.

If you are tempted to break out the biscuits

Usually when temptation strikes, it often isn't about being truly hungry. There may be a different reason behind what is perceived as hunger. When you think you are hungry and it isn't time to eat, check the following:

Am I thirsty? Staying hydrated is essential to well-being but many of us forget to drink enough water. It's amazing what a drink of water can do when you think you are hungry.

Flavoured Waters

Water is essential to good health but many of us struggle to remember to drink enough. I used to keep a large water jug on my desk when I was working, and nowadays I bring a water bottle with me everywhere so that I am drinking lots.

Here are some nice ideas for flavoured waters which help up your quota if you find plain water unappealing:

- lemon slices, rosemary and raspberries
- cucumber, mint and lime
- lemon, ginger and fresh thyme
- blueberry, basil and lemon verbena

Add loads of ice and let your flavours develop a while before enjoying.

Am I tired? Do I need a walk and a quick burst of activity for this to pass? If you tend to have regular slumps, then perhaps log these and try figure out what you can learn from them.

Am I not eating enough, am I eating the wrong foods?

Am I bored? Do I need to change what I am doing, get up from the desk, shake my body out? If you are at a meeting then have a five-minute recess if possible and do a quick trot around the office to wake yourself up.

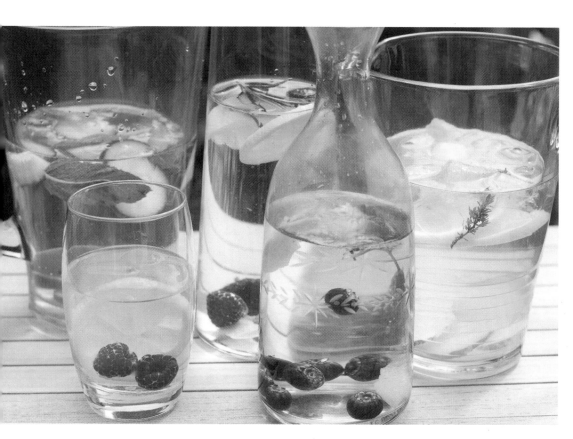

Am I stressed? Often our response to being stressed or unhappy is to reach for food. Recognise if this is your pattern and what you can do to resolve your stresses or unhappiness rather than reaching for food.

Is it in the evening when I am sitting watching TV? This is when mindless eating can occur so watch out for this and keep the unhealthy snacks out of the house to help you break this habit.

Is my energy truly low and therefore I really do need to eat something? Choose something which will feed your body and not put it into a cycle of sugar highs and sugar lows and the resultant continued overeating.

If you do slip up and overdo it

If you have a slip-up and overdo it, the answer is not to starve yourself to try to recoup some of the damage. That isn't good for your body or your mind. The best thing is to pick yourself up again, forgive yourself and go back to the motivation image or vision you worked on before you started. There always is an energy high from starting a new plan and the first few weeks can be easy enough – the gains are becoming apparent, weight is going down, you are feeling a little fitter. It's when that high from feeling great about the idea of your new lifestyle wears off and the motivation is starting to wane because you are a bit tired and don't fancy going to the gym that you need to dig deep in yourself and keep going.

Pull this vision back out again and remind yourself why you decided you were going to get fit and healthy. What is it going to feel like when you have achieved your goal, what will your family and friends say when you make steady progress towards looking and feeling fit and healthy? Think of the future and how much better you are going to feel. Remind yourself of the progress you have already made. Acknowledge that it is OK not to feel totally energised but that it will feel good when you have done it. If you are going to the gym, remind yourself that the hardest part is putting on your gym shorts – once you are there it will be much easier. If you are working out at home, then recruit someone else to keep you going. Friend, partner, child – whoever that person is that you identified in your contingency plan to help.

Reward yourself

Some days I don't feel like working out so I tell myself that when I get home, I'm going to hop into a warm bath and relax for 20 minutes or that I will sit down with a really nice coffee and a book and read for 15 minutes.

Progress: track measurement and celebrate

You should track your goals and record as each week passes and you have done what you said you were going to do. Notice how much better you are starting to feel and acknowledge your success. There is nothing like a bit of success to keep you going! Celebrate it and allow yourself to feel good about what you have achieved. Watch out for your inner critic and any self-talk that might try and scupper the progress you have made. If you tend to struggle with this, try the book by Richard Carson, *Taming your Gremlins* – this is a super little book which gives a lot of insight as to why some of us can allow self-talk to sabotage us.

The basis of our approach to losing or gaining weight is not just about knowing the value of your food intake but also about bringing conscious awareness to eating habits. Bring your attention to how you eat, what you eat and why you eat.

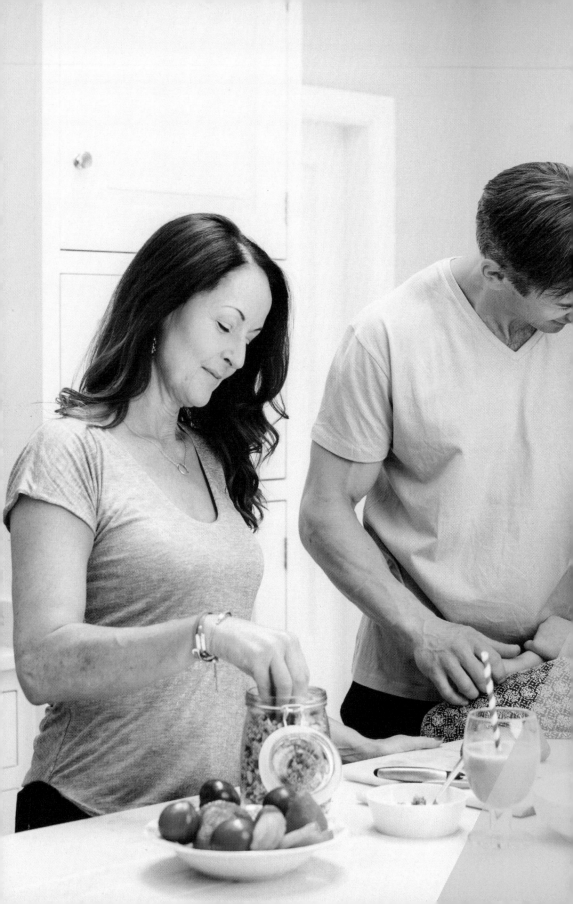

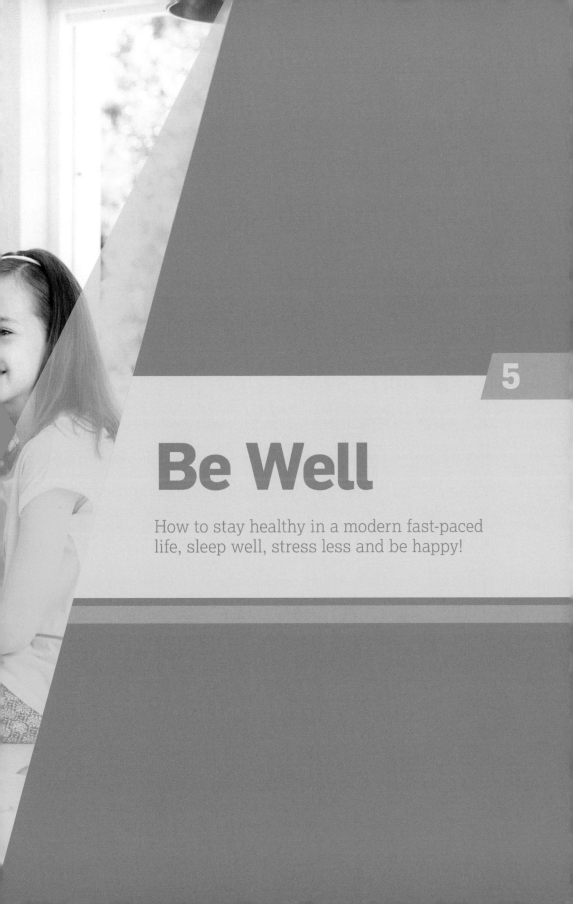

5

Be Well

How to stay healthy in a modern fast-paced life, sleep well, stress less and be happy!

Gráinne's Story

Before I was 32, I buried Ciáran, my first husband, after he died suddenly on a skiing holiday in France. That horrific event was the catalyst for who I am today, where I am today, why I am in the work I now am in and, ultimately, part of what led to this book.

When I was in my teens and early 20s I was too young to fully realise what was really important because I was still growing and learning. I had yet to fall properly in love, my health was good, my career was just starting and I hadn't yet married. Fast forward more than 20 years and all of my life's experiences are part of what makes me and all have taught me something about life and about myself. Now I understand that health, my family and my friends are the most important things in my life.

Growing up, I always loved to cook and loved to help Mum in the kitchen. Being part of a large family meant that was a help, as well as something I got a lot of joy from. I loved cooking for people when the opportunity arose. When I met Ciáran and we started our married life together, we had a lot of fun times and late nights around the kitchen table with friends and family, often ending up with dancing in our sitting room which we nicknamed 'Lansdowne Road' because it had virtually no furniture in it except for a couch and a telly and looked enormous as a result.

I was working away, enjoying my life in the corporate world, having fun, with no real responsibilities as we didn't have kids, had lots of energy and enough money to be able to mostly do the things we wanted.

Early in 1999 I said goodbye to Ciáran as he walked into departures of Dublin Airport for a skiing holiday. I was staying at home – too busy at work to take the time off and just not that into skiing, so I was happy to leave him off to do the thing he loved and see him in a week. But two days later I got a phone call at work that changed my life utterly and completely. Out of the blue and with no warning, Ciáran had died on the side of a mountain in France.

When unimaginable loss barrels towards you, there is no way around it. You can't bypass it; you just have to go through it. I never thought it would get better and couldn't understand how I could still wake up every morning – why hadn't I died from the pain I was feeling? I dreamt endlessly of Ciáran, always the same dream of trying to phone him but not being able to dial his number properly. I used to wake up and, for a millisecond, would have forgotten that he was gone and then the realisation would come crashing in. I thought the pain would never ease. But, gradually, the space between the waves of grief grew wider and I was overcome by it less and less. Little by little, day by day and month by month, the light started to come back.

When we lost our mum not too many years later, I was still grieving for Ciáran and then Mum, too, was gone at a very young age. She had been the pivot around which our family operated. We were all grieving and missing her terribly and following a period of burying myself in work I slowly started to realise that I needed something more from my life and needed to do something totally different from anything I had done before. It seemed natural to me that that would mean something to do with cooking. My mum had taught me to bake and cook and instilled that love in me. I came up with the idea of moving to Rome for a while. I can't honestly tell you where this idea came from, as I had never travelled on my own before. I had been to Rome once and found it hot, busy and a bit unfriendly, so it didn't really make a lot of sense. But something called me there so after a bit of research, I found an apartment and off I went and spent a month living on my own, trying to learn the language and doing cookery classes … in Italian! I landed in that city with not a single word of Italian. Food unites, though, and with a lot of gesturing and miming I found I didn't need the dictionary too much. Romans are wonderfully supportive when they know you are trying to immerse yourself in their city and culture. When I returned home after a month, I knew I had to go back there and, thanks to a very supportive employer, I took time off and back I went. This was just the right thing for me at the time. I had space, no one knew my back story and I started to heal some more. I fell totally in love with Rome and still like to think that I may have been Italian in a previous life!

When I got back to Dublin a friend told me she knew the perfect man for me and asked if I would go on a blind date with Dominic. Having lived on my own in a new city, I felt ready for it so I agreed to dinner and that was the start of a new chapter in my life. Once we got over the hurdle of Dominic thinking that I was a prospective client and not a date, things went well. It wasn't love at first sight but I was very taken by Dominic's kind spirit and we grew closer, fell in love and got married. Thanks to Dominic, I found happiness contentment and love again as well as having our beautiful daughter. Through him I was introduced properly to strength training, something I had never done, although I had always been pretty strong and reasonably sporty.

I spent the majority of my working life in the very high-paced, demanding world of business consulting. I thrived in it, loved the tempo, the variety and challenge of learning and working with new clients. I always cooked to unwind and found my peace and flow when I cooked and fed people.

Becoming a mother, like most, I continued working, juggling the roles of mum, wife and career, and at times struggled to make it all work. Occasionally it became unmanageable, and caused high levels of stress, poor sleep, irritability and feelings of being overwhelmed. So many of us have these kinds of issues in our lives and the struggle is real to get the balance right but there are many valuable tools on how to deal with stress, improve sleep, use meditation, rest and recreation, and keep your life in balance. I so passionately believe in this that when I decided to leave my corporate career I studied Health and Wellness so that I can bring these insights, tools and knowledge to help others and now share in this book. I realise that I am a very resilient person naturally, however, there are many helpful ways to improve how we deal with our very busy lives and lead a life at our full potential. Life for me now is a very happy one but since stresses occur at many points in our life and these can impact our mental health, our happiness, our motivation to eat well and exercise and our physical health, I hope that this chapter will help when the going gets tough and will show how we can manage our lives proactively and be in control of the good days and the bad.

The Fundamentals of Wellness

Most of us, if asked what being well meant, would include feeling happy, coping in times of stress, having good sleep and eating well. But what happens when these aren't going so well and what are some good strategies for getting them back on track again?

Sleep

Sleep trumps everything. While scientists are still discovering precisely why we sleep and what happens when we sleep, we all know that restorative sleep is essential for our physical and mental well-being. Cell regeneration and recovery happens when we sleep, essential cleansing of the byproducts of cell chemical processes happens during sleep, our learning is consolidated and improved when we sleep and memories are examined and filed away as needed – all while we sleep. When we wake up after a good night's sleep, we feel like we can take on the world.

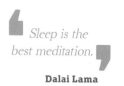

Sleep is the best meditation.

Dalai Lama

If sleep isn't right and doesn't come easily then it can impact all aspects of our life. Poor sleep has been linked to obesity and type 2 diabetes. It can impact heart health and the immune system. It affects our ability to function well at work or school. Waking up still tired makes us irritable and can interfere with our ability to stay calm with our partners, kids and work colleagues. Poor sleep impacts cognitive and physical performance. Elite athletes are now using sleep as one of their weapons to improve performance, and formal studies[1] are emerging that show improvements in sprint time and shooting accuracy when athletes' sleep is improved. Sleep coaches are becoming a part of elite sports management. Fatigue management policies are being developed for large corporations which run round-the-clock shifts or complex industrial processes, to take better care of employees on these shifts and thereby improve safety at work. Poor sleep impacts memory, attention span and reaction time; long-term sleep disorders are known to have a serious negative impact on health and wellness.

In many ways, we don't respect sleep and all it contributes to our well-being. There has been a trend to deride sleep, accompanied by macho reports of how little sleep people can function on. This is not good for us. The invention of the light bulb profoundly changed our sleep patterns and brought with it the ability to run long night shifts but also caused a little-understood but enormous impact on our circadian rhythms. Modern technology is another relatively new factor which is having a detrimental effect on our natural sleeping patterns, and we are sleeping less and less. In the last decade with the rise of mobile phones, we are disrupting our circadian rhythms with overexposure to their blue light late at night. Our children are being raised for a lifetime of bad sleeping habits unless we do something about it now. It is an easy trap to fall into – hanging onto our phones or tablets by the bed or in the

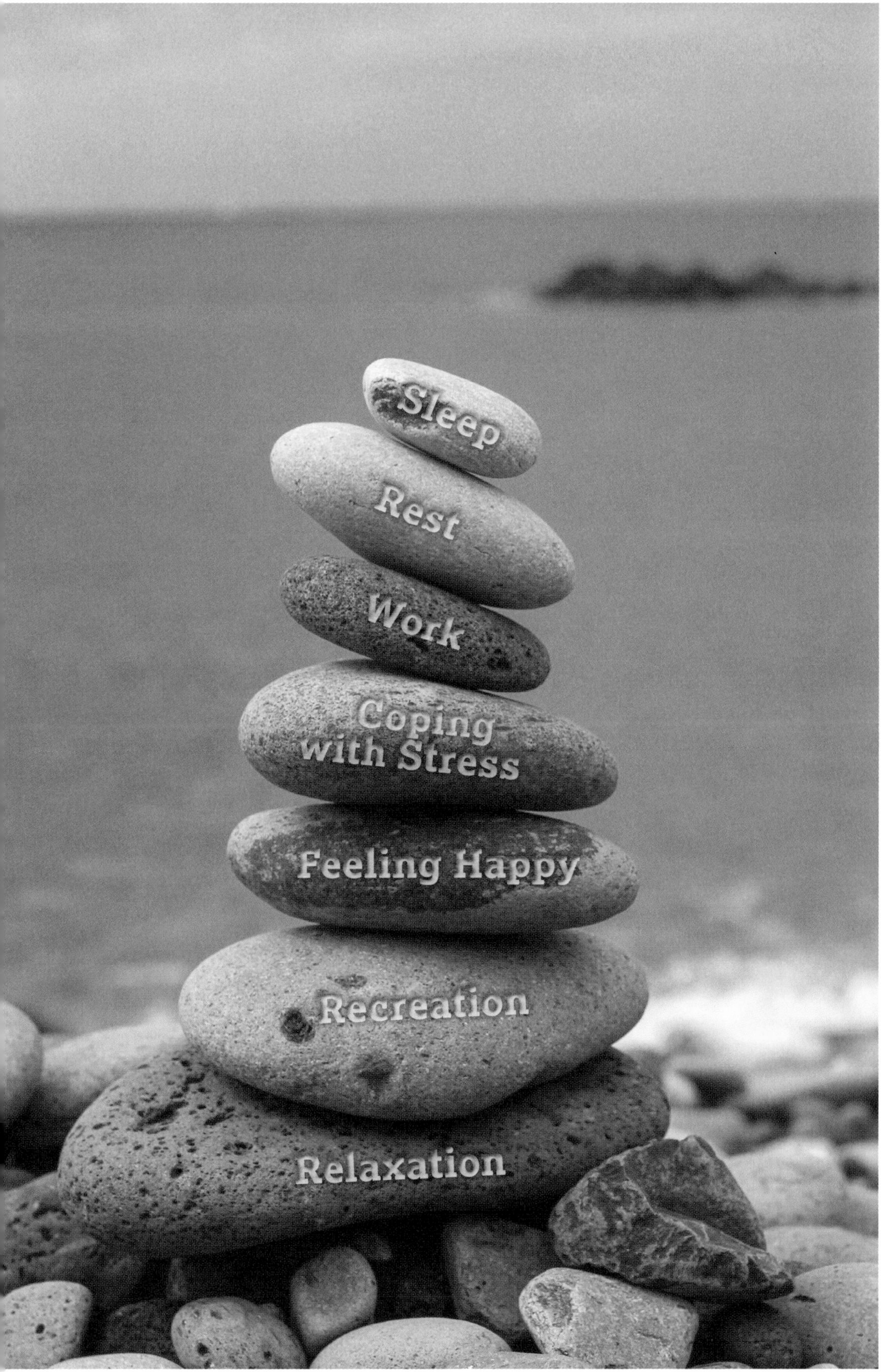

hours before bedtime. The harsh lighting emitted from these devices tell our pineal gland not to produce melatonin, which is the wrong message when we want to power down and go to sleep. Supressing melatonin (which I like to call the lullaby hormone) is extremely disruptive to our bodies at night and essentially your body is no longer being instructed to sleep. I love my bed and midweek can be found curled up with a good book by 10.30 p.m. because that is what works for me. I don't function well on less than seven and a half hours' sleep so I make sure I get to bed in time to have that.

It is true that occasional periods of bad sleep can happen, especially if we are having a particularly stressful time, whether that be in work or our personal life. If it is a temporary blip, there are many things you can do to help improve sleep. However, chronic stress can impact your hormones and therefore your sleep – you are not getting appropriate recovery and it is not good for health to be sleep-deprived for too long. If this is the case, seek medical or sleep-professional help to check that there is no undiagnosed root cause.

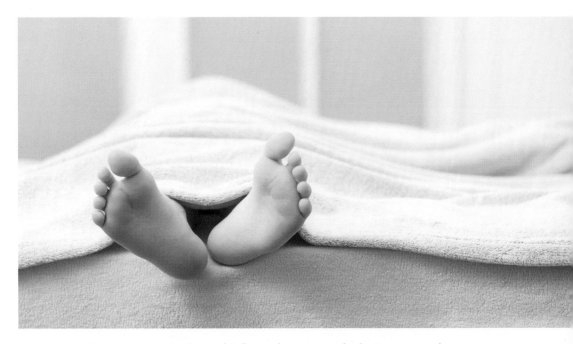

Here are some tips which are known to help improve sleep:

Create a sanctuary
Make your room a place where only sleep, relaxation or sex happens. Get rid of the TV, clear away clutter and pick any stuff off your bed – there is just no pleasure to be had if you have to clear the bed before you jump into it.

Get rid of all electronic devices from your room and power down from using phones, tablets, etc., at least 30 minutes before bedtime. If they are downstairs then, if you wake up in the middle of the night, you won't be tempted to check your email. Ensure your room is dark but allow a little natural light in to help wake you up naturally and don't have your room too warm – a cooler temperature is better for sleep and find a mattress and pillow you enjoy sleeping on.

Have a wind-down routine

Purposefully make time to switch off before bed so that there is a wind-down process to help prepare the body for bed and let the mind know that it is time to start relaxing. We always make a pot of peppermint tea about an hour before bed. This helps slow us down and is our signal to the body and mind that bedtime is soon. Find out what wind-down works for you: perhaps have a bath or write out the 'To Do' list for the next day.

Work out your optimum amount of sleep, which for most of us is seven to nine hours, and try go to bed at the same time and get up at the same time every day, in order to achieve that. All the latest studies show that timing trumps being tired; regularly going to bed too late results in sleep debt and you won't sleep long enough to catch up properly.

Prepare everything you need for the next day the night before: clothes, bag, school and work lunches.

Try some sleep aids

Deep, relaxing breathing for a few minutes before getting into bed is very helpful to help slow the mind from its endless cycle of thought after thought. There is a very strong link between mindfulness through meditation exercises and our wellness and long-term health. Meditation is an enormously powerful tool in our arsenal to improve our sleep quality as well as our ability to handle stress. When we can't sleep, it is essentially because we can't persuade our brain to stop being our brain and so it keeps on thinking and thinking and we stay awake. Meditation will help slow our thoughts and enables our brain to shut up!

Magnesium is good for improving sleep. There are lots of studies emerging about the improvements in sleep quality through increasing the levels of magnesium in your diet. It is found in leafy greens, such as spinach and kale, so get cracking on those recipes in this book. It is also depleted by sugar and alcohol, so think about whether you need to address your consumption of those. In addition, sweating during exercise depletes it. Epsom salts in the bath are a great passive way to get some in (as well as helping you to relax before bed). While the ideal is to get all you need from food, it is not always possible and, if your sleep quality is chronically bad, it can be worth checking with your GP whether you might have a magnesium deficiency. We use a liquid spray of magnesium citrate and find it beneficial.

Finally, watch your intake of alcohol and caffeine: while the benefits of a small amount of alcohol are known, too much is bad for our sleep. This is because, while it may cause you to feel sleepy initially, it can block REM sleep and the quality of our sleep suffers. Similarly, caffeine is not good for you close to bedtime and many studies conclude that you should not have caffeine in a six-hour window before bed. I love coffee – it would be one of my desert island luxuries but I rarely have it after 2 p.m. If I'm silly enough to drink it late at night, say when eating out, usually when the soporific effects of any wine wear off, I end up wide awake at 4 a.m. and so it's just not worth it.

Morning routine and intention setting

When you wake, give yourself a minute just before you start to get ready, and set some intentions for the day. I swear by this – even if it is just to try and do a little better than the previous day if I have been a bit grumpy. This works well to help set my mindset for the day. I tell myself it is going to be a good day, that I am going to have some fun, that I'm going to help my daughter today – whatever it is you want to achieve for the day. Studies have shown that framing a positive point of view actually helps us to feel happier – expecting a good day rather than expecting a bad day.

In the months after Ciáran died, I used this tool. When I woke up, I used to tell myself that all I had to do was get out of bed and get to work. It helped me enormously because it didn't set too many expectations, just a small task. I had an enormously supportive family and group of friends, including in work, and once there I found that I was able to bury myself in work, which I had always derived pleasure and a sense of achievement from, and it helped me forget about this awful reality just for a while. If I had a really bad day I was able to reach out to the people around me and they helped me through it.

I didn't sleep well for a long time but I accepted that this was normal and wasn't worried about it. The same goes for you – there will be times in your life when you won't sleep well and will feel stressed, excited or upset. Bringing your awareness to these and trying some of the actions listed above will help.

Happiness

Years ago, I worked with a wonderful Spanish man who always used to say that when he woke up he made the decision to be happy and have a good day. He was always very cheerful and was a lovely positive person to be around. (You know who you are, Pedro!) You may read this and think, 'I can't just decide to be happy' and I'm the first to admit that being Irish means that cynicism is in our DNA, but it does work – really! Large numbers of studies now show that you can reframe your thinking. The positive choice to 'Be Happy' can absolutely help make us feel happy.

There are studies emerging to understand what the factors are that keep us happy, and they all show a clear pattern of essential but simple elements which, when we work to include

> *Happiness is not something ready made. It comes from our own actions.*
>
> **Dalai Lama**

them in our lives, increase our happiness, our feelings of belonging and our overall well-being. This is not an encouragement to pursue hedonistic feelings purely for the sake of them but to make the concerted effort to cultivate positive emotions. They make us more resilient and become a bank we can draw on during bad times.

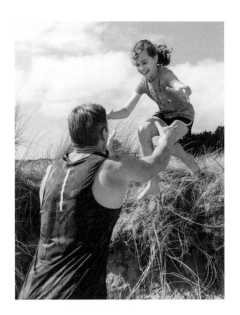

The Five Ways to Well-being.²

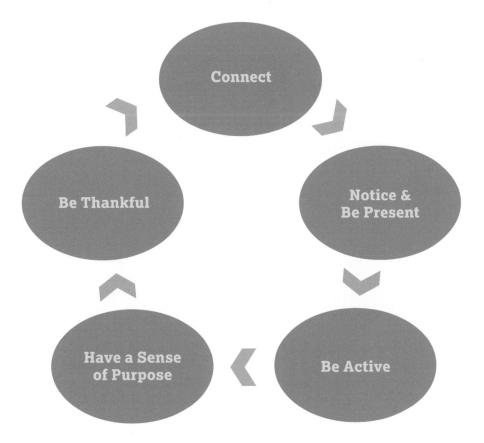

Connect

Good relationships keep us living longer, happier and healthier so the reminder is to nurture our relationships – especially keep them going when times are busy, as this is when you need your friends most but are most likely to drop them. Remember: it's quality, not quantity, and it's not on Facebook but in real life. Feeling lonely is bad for your health. It is known that the body has an adverse biological response to loneliness so don't let being busy or being stressed trump efforts to connect with friends and family. That isn't the same as being alone – time out is good for us, too. I love curling up with a good book, a habit I inherited from my mum. She always said that you would never be lonely when you had a book. She was so right – when I started going on holidays on my own, I always felt OK about going to restaurants by myself when I had something to read. I had something to keep me occupied and I met people through conversations struck up over being asked about what I was reading.

> *Friendships double joy and cut grief in half.*
>
> **Francis Bacon**

Good, close relationships buffer us from the 'slings and arrows' of growing old.[3] They are good for our health and well-being. Our 'bonding' hormone, Oxytocin, helps us want to spend time with people, which will help reduce our stress. Sometimes we withdraw when we are stressed, thinking ourselves too busy to spend time with friends. Spending time with people will help us respond well to stressful times so don't withdraw. Work hard, even in busy times, to cultivate and keep your group of close friends and family – there is nothing like a good laugh with friends to help you feel good.

Notice and be present

Seeing what is around us in the world, in nature, and happening at this very minute helps us get rid of any pattern of dwelling on the past. Enjoy life as it is happening now: the chats with family, the walk to work, the glass of wine with friends. Living in the past, going over what we said yesterday or what someone said to us, is exhausting, steals our energy and is a waste of precious time. This includes comparing ourselves to others, which really is the thief of joy. In these days of perfectly curated Instagram images, it could be easy to believe that everyone else has a perfect, beautiful life. The reality is that most people are going through the same joys and challenges as you are and no one's life is perfect in reality. Comparison has a detrimental effect on our happiness and can make us feel inadequate. Silence it by recognising it as comparison talk which serves no purpose other than to impact your happiness.

To quote a favourite 1980s movie: 'Spend a little more time trying to make something of yourself and a little less time trying to impress people.' (*The Breakfast Club*)

Be active

Be active – walk, run, cycle, go to the gym, do yoga – whatever exercise floats your boat will help you feel good. Find the thing you really enjoy and make time for it and your feelings of well-being and happiness will improve. Get outside into nature for a sense of being connected to the earth we live on.

Have a sense of purpose

A sense of purpose to our life is one of the key aspects to wellness and living fully. For some of us, our sense of purpose is our job or our hobby, especially when we can immerse ourselves completely in it. The state we achieve when we do an activity and get totally in the zone, are really enjoying it and our minds don't wander around, is called being 'in flow'. This 'flow' means we are completely engaged in what we are doing. I know many people who talk about things they loved when they were younger or when they had more time. If you can identify the activity that gives you this feeling of flow and do it as your job or your hobby, it can give you your sense of purpose, so cultivate it for a rewarding, happier life. If you aren't sure what your sense of purpose is, consider what it is that makes you tick: is it learning something new, is it helping others and contributing to society, or something more modest? My own sense of purpose comes from cooking and feeding others. I love people around my table and the connections made around food.

Be thankful

Being thankful seems to be one of the buzz phrases of recent years, but the concept of gratitude has been around for a long time. Consider the concept of giving thanks, the way people used to say Grace before meals, where a family would join together and say thanks for the food they were about to receive. Studies show that people who actively notice what they are grateful for report feeling happier and more content. The act of gratitude brings our awareness to the things we have in our life that are good and is strongly associated with feelings of well-being, less likelihood of being depressed as well as being resilient in times of challenge.

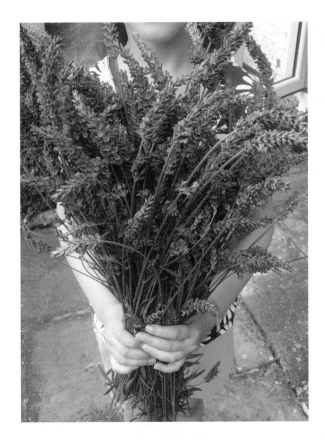

All these habits serve to cultivate our feelings of satisfaction with our lives and our sense of happiness. It doesn't mean that we should just bury feelings of sadness or pretend that we aren't having a bad time; it means that we make efforts to improve our situation and our happiness by proactively managing it. It gives us the tools to be in control of the good days and the bad days. If you are feeling low and it isn't passing, reach out for help: help from friends or family, or your local GP if needed, as you may be suffering from clinical depression. If you are clinically depressed, you will need a professional to work alongside you and help you recover. For me, when I was grieving, it wasn't an illness that could be treated, but clinical depression is, so get help and don't suffer alone.

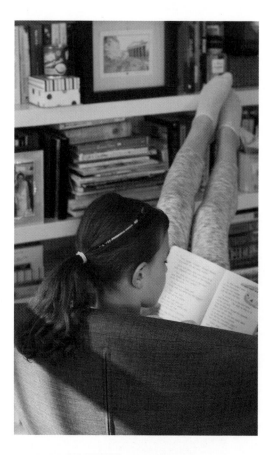

Stress

Our stress response is the body's way of coping with danger and is vital when danger occurs. The big problem in our modern life is that we are turning on our stress response chronically and continually, triggered by both acute and non-acute emergencies and worries. These can range from the everyday pressures of life right through to dramatic life-changing events such as death or illness in the family, moving house, breakdown of a relationship, divorce, or changing or losing one's job.

The right level of stress is a good thing and a remarkable aid to get things done but unmanageable levels of stress can undo us if we are not recovering properly. Key to this is ensuring that we can recognise our own stress triggers, develop a way of responding appropriately to those triggers and allow for recovery and recreation to ensure that we have balance in our life and thus build our stress resilience.

At its simplest, stress is a thought or thoughts in response to something happening to us, real or imagined, which then gives rise to physical symptoms in our body. These include heart beating faster as it pumps more oxygen around your body, glucose being quickly shunted to your cells to get ready to provide energy and your senses becoming heightened. Your immunity in the short term is improved and some other body systems become less important as you get ready to deal with the immediate crisis. There are a variety of very complex hormonal interactions involved in these processes which should return to balance when the 'danger' passes but when we are continually stressed and chronically turning on this stress response, these hormones can get out of whack and have a very significant adverse effect on our physical and mental health. The list is long and includes impaired cognitive performance, problems with sleep, cardiovascular problems from elevated blood pressure, a reduction in our immune response in the long term, blood sugar imbalances and potentially type 2 diabetes. Decreased serotonin increases the risk of depression and has been associated with increased abdominal fat, which is associated with higher levels of heart problems and stroke. Just reading this is enough to start the worry process!

There is a huge amount written about the negative impact of stress on our lives and I have experienced significant periods in my life where I was traumatically stressed as part of the grief process but also later on in life when I suffered a lot of work-related stress. This was a very new experience to me, one I didn't even recognise. Previously, stress had served me well and I had been functioning effectively during very busy, pressurised periods of work. However, when I become a parent, I no longer had as much personal freedom for my own rest and recovery and since I wasn't very good at recognising that I was stressed, I also wasn't very good at actively working to manage it.

To develop a good stress response, it is vital to learn how to recognise it, how to understand it, how to respond to it and how important rest and recreation are in balancing life's stresses. Often, the external factors that cause stress can't be controlled but how we respond and our patterns of behaviour in the face of stress are very important in managing it to prevent its ill effects, unhappiness and adverse health impacts. Essentially, we need to make stress our friend and not our enemy. Finding the way to deal with stress that works for you will help you retain your health and wellness. If you suffer from chronic stress, poor sleep and/or low levels of anxiety, I implore you to continue to try to solve the problem. If nothing else is working, perhaps consider a visit to your GP to see if further investigation or a counsellor might be needed for you.

How to reduce anxiety

This is a good exercise for when you start to feel stressed or your anxiety levels rise:

- The first very useful thing to do is remind yourself that these symptoms are useful to you – they are your body's way of getting you ready for something important. These actually facilitate performance. If you are just about to do a presentation or an important work interview, harness these feelings to your advantage. Instead of feeling overwhelmed by them, tell yourself that these are good feelings that mean you are ready to perform. Energy is being directed to the right place: my heart is racing because I am excited!

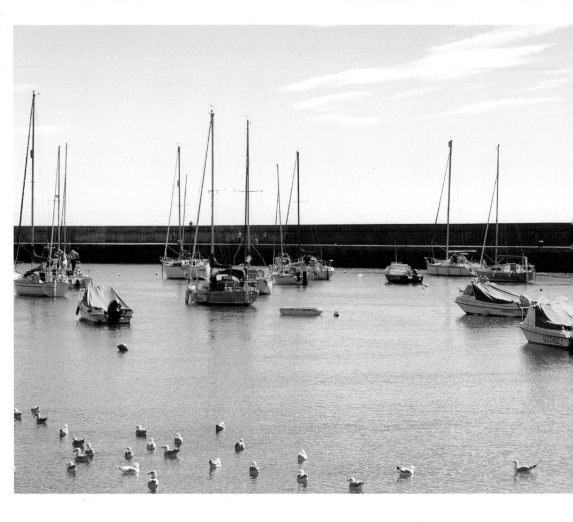

- Do a quick body scan and see what is tight – usually the neck, shoulders and jaw. Relax them and then slow everything down by taking a few slow, controlled, deep belly breaths to help you calm yourself down and give yourself some space before you begin.

- If you are in an interaction with someone, just pause before action and examine your thoughts and decide how best to respond. Ask yourself: am I jumping to conclusions here, what is the perspective of the other person in this interaction and what will serve me best when I respond?

- If you can, take a five-minute break and get some fresh air and reflect on how you are feeling and what you can do to help yourself in that immediate moment. Just taking that break and slowing down will help.

If you can manage the source of stress then you can proactively work to relieve it.

Identify the cause of stress

Identify what causes the stress in your life. What are the triggers that cause a pattern of stressful thoughts arising? We can't control what goes on externally but we can control ourselves and our own actions, so figure out if these contribute to stress arising. Are you always late? If so, you need to sort out your time management. Do you leave everything to the last minute? If so, you need to get organised.

Do you say yes to everything and therefore get bogged down with a huge, unmanageable workload which keeps you awake at night worrying about? Do you occasionally say no, only to suffer guilty feelings? We all like helping people. We are encouraged to be helpful at school, growing up, in family life, etc., but it can be useful to examine whether you are the person who says yes all the time and is inclined to get overworked and perhaps even a bit walked on as a result. This can be a tricky one to change because you can get pushback from work or even family who are more used to you always saying yes. I'm not suggesting you start being completely unhelpful but make an effort to gain a good balance so that you are not overworked and taken for granted. Before you say yes, examine what might need to be dropped, delayed or not done at all. If it's at work and your boss has an urgent request, outline what you currently have on your priority list and negotiate what needs to be reprioritised, delegated or delayed.

Are you a perfectionist?

It can be useful to examine whether you are a perfectionist and need to stop sacrificing good enough on the altar of perfection. Being a perfectionist is not a good thing at all: perfectionists are hard to work with, difficult to have on a team and tend to waste time on activities that don't add value. Excellence is not the same as perfection – we don't suggest you should do a bad job but take some time for introspection to recognise if perfectionism is a trait of yours that you need to change.

At work, do you need to learn to delegate more? And if you do delegate, can you allow and cope with the fact that things will be done 'not your way'? One of my colleagues at work used to tell me how his other half asked him to help with the ironing and then used to stand over him and watch and critique how he did it! It can be helpful to have a trusted mentor at work whom you can talk to and get advice from about what is going on: someone who can give you a different perspective, maybe spot something about your own behaviour that could be making the situation, and therefore the stress, worse.

Examine and take the best of the behaviours of people who don't seem to suffer from stress

It is really interesting to take two people and put them in the same 'stressful' situation and see how different their reactions are. I had a hellish client once and really struggled with the situation. One of my colleagues had no issue and did not worry about it in the same way I did. I asked them how they didn't appear to suffer and learnt a lot listening to them. They explained that there was no changing this client: their culture was to be this way, therefore they would do their best for them but accepted that this client would still rant and rave so they were not going to lose sleep over them. I had been taking it personally but it just wasn't personal. This was a huge lesson for me in dealing with external stress.

Have you the boss from hell?

I have been really lucky and worked for some amazing people but I have met one or two hellish individuals along the way. Chances are, if you are under pressure from a hellish boss, they are as well, from whoever is above them. Learn what your manager's stress conditions and derailment factors are and figure out what the best tactic is to deal with them. If there are people who seem to be able to work well with them, study what they do and see if there is something you can do to improve matters. And always make sure your work isn't one of the reasons why your boss kicks off – high-quality work speaks for itself.

Identify what's going on

Is it an external situation that needs to be resolved? This could be a relationship issue, or a row with a parent or sibling, or money worries. Making the decision to do something positive to resolve what you have been worrying about can really help with the resulting stress … as long as you move beyond making the decision into the action stage. I have learnt to ask myself what are the one or two positive actions I can take to start to resolve this thing I am stressing about and then write down what I am going to do and when I am going to do it. Even the act of taking the time to examine what is causing your stress can help bring clarity and resolve.

It's not personal

Not everything that happens to us is personal and it can be a human habit to go over and over in our minds what has happened and remind ourselves how upset, cross or sad that made us feel. This perpetual cycle of rekindling anger is not healthy. Letting go of these feelings and realising that sometimes this stuff just happens for no reason is incredibly freeing and can help reduce feelings of stress.

A good day starts the night before

Before you go to bed, make a list of the must-dos for the day. Get everything ready so there is no stress in the morning. Try and get up 15 minutes early. This will allow you to be a little more leisurely getting to work. When I started working I was also learning to drive so I used to go in at the crack of dawn because I didn't want to meet any other cars on the road. I developed a habit of being an early bird (in at 7 a.m.!). I'm not saying you should go to work that early but having some time before the office or shopfloor starts to hum is great for getting the day planned. I used to make myself a nice coffee and sit down and plan the day. It also gives you time to say hello properly to people and have a chat with your colleagues and really connect with others.

Let your brain solve your problems

If you have a problem, give it over to your brain to solve it. When I started out as a business analyst I would have errors in my coding and couldn't for the life of me figure out what was wrong. I used to go to bed and would wake in the middle of the night and realise where the error was and how to fix it. It was an incredible experience to realise that my brain had been solving the problem for me. Our brains are amazing, so when you have a problem to solve, just let your brain do its thing and you will be surprised at what it can resolve for you as part of good sleep routines.

Keep a journal and pencil beside your bed – if you find you are waking up with a racing mind, jot down what's bothering you and then tell yourself to let it go, that it will be there for you in the morning. If getting back to sleep is a problem, try deep breathing: in for the count of five, hold your breath for a second or two and then breathe deeply out for the count of five, focusing on your breath as you do this. Again, magnesium is helpful to the body in this mind-racing scenario.

Real worries

Stress can often be about imagined worries but real worries, such as money worries, fear of losing your job or worrying about keeping a roof over your head, are naturally huge causes of stress. These worries have a detrimental impact on health and well-being. Of course we worry about these things and it would be trite to say 'try not to worry'. Get all the help you can to manage these circumstances, for example, from your local Citizens Information Centre, or other agencies set up to help people. If you are dealing with these worries then efforts to help calm your mind using meditation, getting as good sleep as you can, eating as well as possible, and time outside in nature can only help you.

Mindfulness and meditation

There is a huge body of evidence showing the link between being mindful or meditating and stress reduction. Taking time to connect with your thoughts and doing some simple meditative breathing will help slow your mind down and your body's feelings of stress – allowing you to find some 'me' time. Our brain wants to do its job, which essentially involves lots of thinking. When this thinking never stops and you get caught in a spiral of poor sleep and feeling stressed, it's time to teach your brain how to switch off. The benefits of taking ten minutes to walk around the block, breathing in and down into your belly and out slowly (as described in the Move Well chapter) is very calming in stressful times and you can do it anywhere. Developing a meditation habit is one of the best weapons in dealing with stress in your life. If you aren't sure where to start, there are loads of books and apps to help. Apps like the Mind Space App, Calm App and Oprah & Deepak's 21-day meditation experience are a good introduction, as is Jon Kabat-Zinn's book on mindfulness-based stress reduction (MBSR), *Mindfulness for Beginners*, which is known all over the world. The techniques are offered by hospitals, and health and wellness organisations, especially in the USA but becoming more common here in Europe too. This isn't new, though the technology available is, and it really works.

Exercise

Any form of exercise is excellent for stress reduction and as well as keeping us fitter, stronger and more mobile, it helps us cope with busier periods in life, helps us to sleep better and relax. Oftentimes it can be the first thing that goes out the window when we are very busy at work or feeling stressed but you should do your utmost not to let that happen. Keep to your planned workouts, but make them shorter if time is really constrained. Exercise will help reduce the elevated levels of stress hormones in the body as well as producing feel-good hormones; it will help you feel better, relax more, sleep better and ultimately feel less stressed. Don't overdo it though – it's not about beating yourself up in the gym. This will only layer physical stress on top of mental and/or emotional stress, so remember to treat yourself with kindness when you are exercising.

Eat right

Now more than ever is the time to eat lots of fresh fruit and vegetables to help nourish your body. Loading up with processed food will bring sugar lows, make you feel awful and exacerbate the stress. Skipping meals because you are too busy to eat is the quick way to illness. No matter how busy life and work are, you should take proper breaks and ensure you aren't going too long without nourishing food.

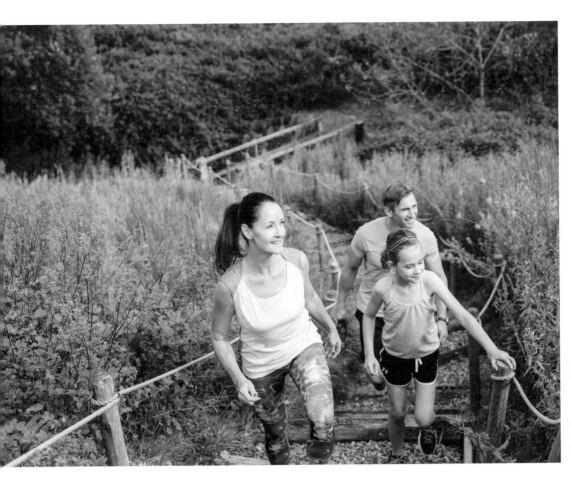

Be kind to yourself

There will always be a huge 'To Do' list. There will never be nothing that needs doing. However, sometimes you just need to say 'sod it' and take some time out to relax. I always ask clients to consider whether something is urgent and important, and if not, to take it a bit easier on themselves and just take some time to recharge.

Talk and be social

When things get stressful, it's good to talk about it and share what is happening. If you are working and things get crazy, teamwork can improve if people can acknowledge that it is a bit stressful for the moment. Making the effort to connect with people, whether over a coffee or a quick walk, can help make feelings of stress more manageable and less isolating. Bonding in this way helps! If your personal life is stressing you, don't bottle it up: find someone who can lend an ear and encourage you to keep your rest and recreation, exercise and eat well to offset your stressful feelings.

Time outside

Getting fresh air and feeling connected to nature is essential to well-being. Remember how good you feel after a walk on the beach or in the woods. Make time to reconnect your body to the earth we live on. At work, if you have loads of meetings, try make some of them walking-outside meetings. In this way, you will up your activity, get fresh air and have the meeting you need. Winner all round!

Recreation as your stress antidote

Recreation. The meaning of this word has been lost in modern times but if you think of it as two words – 're' and 'creation' – the purpose of recreation and its role in balancing stress becomes more obvious. Your own outlet to find inner peace is essential to balance stress in the body. For some it is gardening, walking, reading, cooking, art – whatever it is that you used to love to do until you got too busy in life is that essential activity which will help you recharge your batteries and manage your busy life with energy and feeling happy, not stressed and harried. Find the time for what helps you be in the moment, centres you and makes you feel happy and this will act as an antidote to stress.

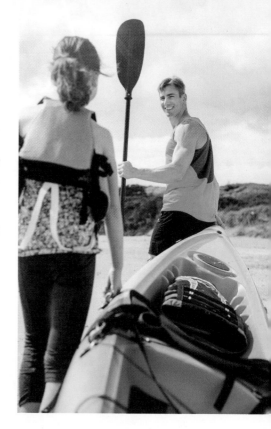

Set boundaries

We all should have boundaries, particularly on our working life so that it doesn't all blur into one endless day. Know what those are for you, such as when you switch off the laptop, the phone, weekend working, etc., and ensure you have some regular, predictable downtime. Even if it is hellish at work and an all-shoulders-to-the-wheel time of year, you should still try and schedule downtime to rest and recharge. Building resilience to stress isn't just about surviving it; it is about recharging and renewing so that you can thrive.

A final word on reducing stress is not to let these tips become a stick to beat yourself with. Find the few things that really work for you and stick with them. There is no point becoming stressed because you haven't had time to do all of these – look for the balance in everything and be kind to yourself.

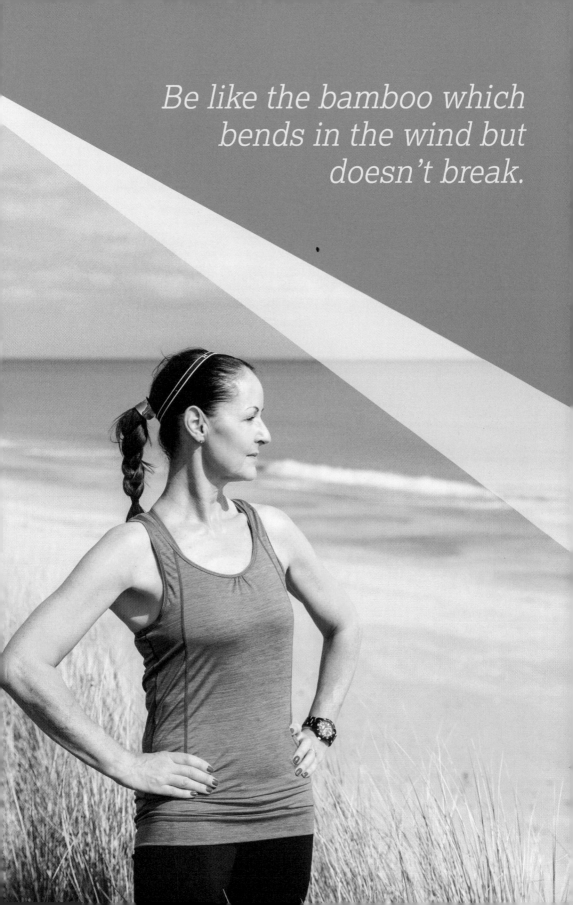

Be like the bamboo which bends in the wind but doesn't break.

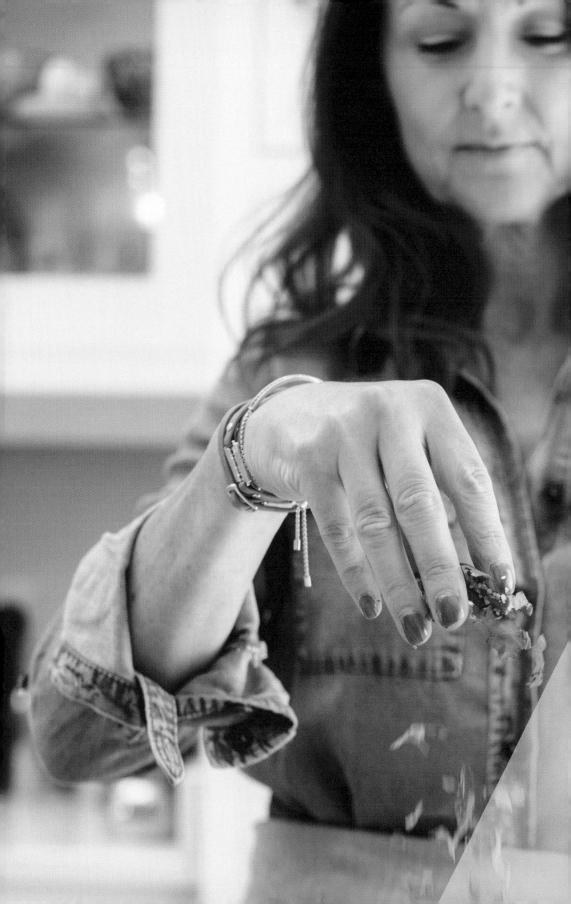

6

Recipes

Lots of delicious recipes help you find
balance and eat in a better way

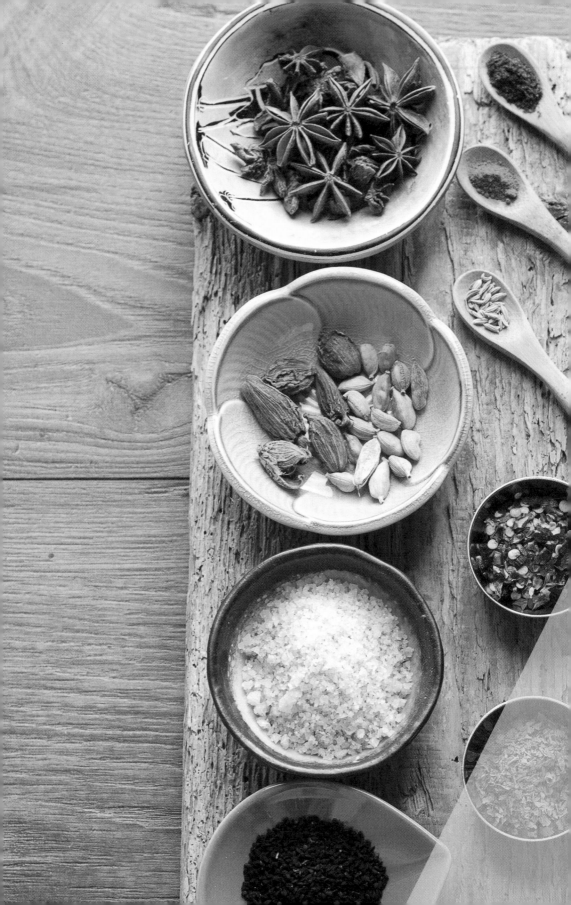

If we eat at the table with family and friends, conversation is better and connections are real.

Food is much more than fuel. It's not about finding the perfect post-workout window to get your protein in or cheat meals earned by starving yourself all week so you can sit down and dig into a huge bowl of ice cream, cakes or chocolate. Food is so much more than that, it's pleasure, nature's gift to us, it is the opportunity to sit down with friends and loved ones to truly connect. This is where the food philosophy of the fitness industry has gone so badly wrong, thinking of food as the enemy to be controlled. Food is our friend to be loved and respected. We are old school when it comes to food because we fundamentally believe we should eat and enjoy real food, just not too much of it.

This is the food we like to eat. None of the recipes are complicated and while they don't take ages to prepare, we believe it takes time to develop a bit of flavour so if you are simmering something on the hob, give it time; your food will be all the better for it. I was taught to season, and old habits die hard, so I always use salt and pepper in my recipes especially where there are no herbs or other spices. I know we need to watch our salt intake but I like the extra lift a little seasoning adds. It takes food from 'grand' to 'really lovely'. It is up to you, though, so if you don't like to add salt or pepper, don't feel compelled to. I understand the health worries of excess salt in food but if you are buying your meat, fish, and veg raw and unprepared, you are avoiding all the salt-laden processed food offered in packaged dinners. Unless you have been ordered onto a low-salt diet, you shouldn't have any concerns.

You also won't find any recipes for porridge or pancakes here. Firstly, you couldn't pay me enough to eat porridge – admittedly I was force-fed it as a child (not literally, but you get the picture) but when it came back up I was never offered it again. As for pancakes, they are a regular weekend breakfast in the house and even our daughter knows how to throw them together, so I didn't bother including them here.

Recipe nutrition data

The nutrition information provides an approximate breakdown of calories per portion, as well as protein, carbohydrates, fat and fibre. The information is useful as a base for calculating what you are taking in per portion size rather than being scientifically exact. This is because ingredients vary when you cook the recipe. Your medium chicken breast might be considered large by someone else – and the same goes for fruit and veg. We have provided numbers of portions for each of the recipes so if you eat more than one portion, remember to recalculate the calories taken in!

The skinny on sugar

Sugar rightly has a bad reputation and overconsumption can cause havoc with our insulin levels, leading to increased risk of type 2 diabetes. Our body is capable of handling small amounts of sugar. The fundamental problem with sugar is that people can't be trusted around it and a diet high in sugar is a constant test of your willpower. Sugar is something of a Trojan horse. The high you get from its overconsumption is always followed by a sugar crash, adverse health impacts and a craving for more.

The global rise in obesity can be linked not just to sugar but to all foods because we are consuming ever increasing amounts of calories on a daily basis, sadly more and more of it from processed foods and less and less of it from fruits, vegetables, fish, meat, beans and good grains. The so-called healthy sugars proposed as an alternative to our run-of-the-mill white stuff still contain significant calories and should be treated as sugar.

So, what about these alternatives and how should they be used ... apart from in moderation!

Regular white sugar contains 394kcals per 100g

Agave nectar

This is the sap of the Mexican agave plant, touted as healthy due to its low GI (or Glycaemic Index, the number which reflects the effect a food has on a person's glucose or blood sugar level); however, this is not something widely used in our kitchen. It is primarily fructose and we don't like it or recommend its use as a sugar replacement because it is metabolised in the liver and converted to fat as part of digestion.

Contains 310kcals per 100g

Blackstrap molasses

This is the syrup produced when sugar cane is processed to make sugar. It has a very robust flavour (read: not entirely pleasant), and I'm speaking from experience as I have memories of being lined up as a kid to have my daily dose of it and trying to run out to the garden to find somewhere to hide it. It contains some vitamins and minerals if well produced. I use this when I make brown bread as a spoon of it adds a nice flavour, but I don't use it for much else.

Contains 290kcal per 100g

Coconut sugar

Depressingly expensive, this is the sap of the coconut palm and is less processed than its white sugar relative. I love to bake with it because of the complex caramel flavours it has. It also contains inulin, a type of fibre which enables slower digestion.

Contains 387kcal per 100g

Honey

Produced by bees, it tastes according to the bees' diet. It can have amino acids and minerals, depending on production. I love to use it in marinades or for sweetening up dressings.

Contains 300kcal per 100g

Maple syrup

This is from maple tree sap. Beware of products masquerading as it and look for 100 per cent pure maple. This is also depressingly expensive. I will use this for baking, though not for cakes for any nice occasion, just for flapjacks or cookies.

Contains 261kcal per 100g

Raw sugar (demerara, turbinado, brown)

This is the same as white sugar but is slightly less processed and contains molasses and hence more complex flavours. If you are buying it, make sure that's what you are getting and not coloured white sugar.

Contains 380kcal per 100g

Stevia

This is a natural sweetener made from the leaves of the stevia plant. It has no calories despite being sweeter than sugar. It is highly processed and has a bitter aftertaste. It also doesn't caramelise and I don't consider it suitable at all as a sugar replacement for baking. Fine to use if you really need to have sugar in your tea or coffee.

Contains 0 calories

Bottom line – sugars are sugars and low consumption is key.

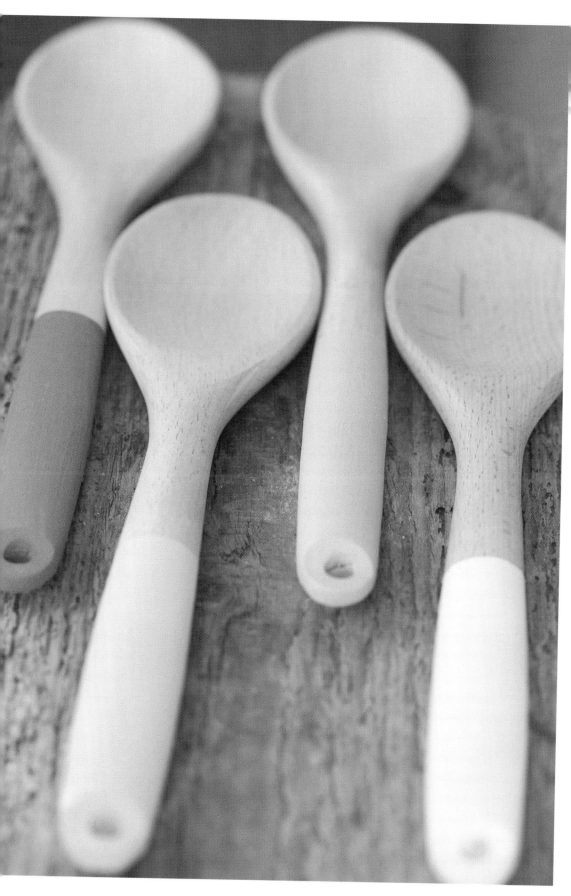

The Recipes

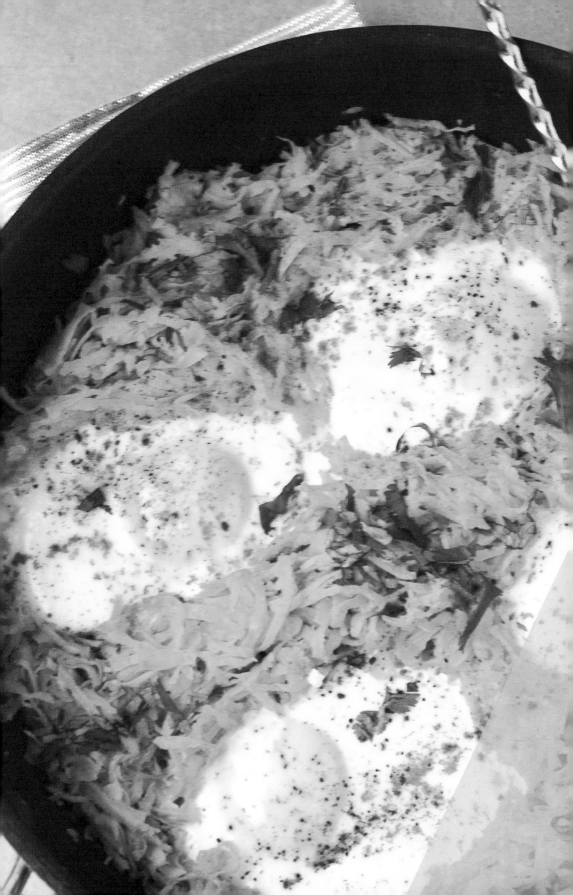

Breakfasts

Not everyone likes to eat breakfast and in some cases, it is the right decision. We get that. We believe only children should have to have breakfast; otherwise, if you believe you work best eating later, then don't have it. There are many studies on the benefit of intermittent fasting so if you don't need brekkie and you aren't overweight, sluggish or tired then I would suggest it works for you. As an exception, if you are going to the gym first thing or doing a workout, then it is good to eat something beforehand. If you haven't been eating breakfast and have been feeling tired, then chances are you might need it, so have a think about whether your no-breakfast habit is really right for you.

I have quite a few recipes for eggs here. They are basically our desert-island food – we go through huge amounts of them each week, whether simply boiled or more effort put in for weekend brunch-style family breakfasts. We also do a fair bit of juicing – not always during the week but almost always at the weekend. I try and have one third of the contents as vegetables when it comes to juices. I don't overdo the green – to me it just tastes like I'm eating grass so I need to have a good bit of fruit. I often start the day with a glass of hot water and lemon, as well as some apple cider vinegar – a small 10ml shot with a glass of water at the ready (because, to be honest, it's a bit harsh on the tastebuds. Dominic can neck it but I'm not that hardy).

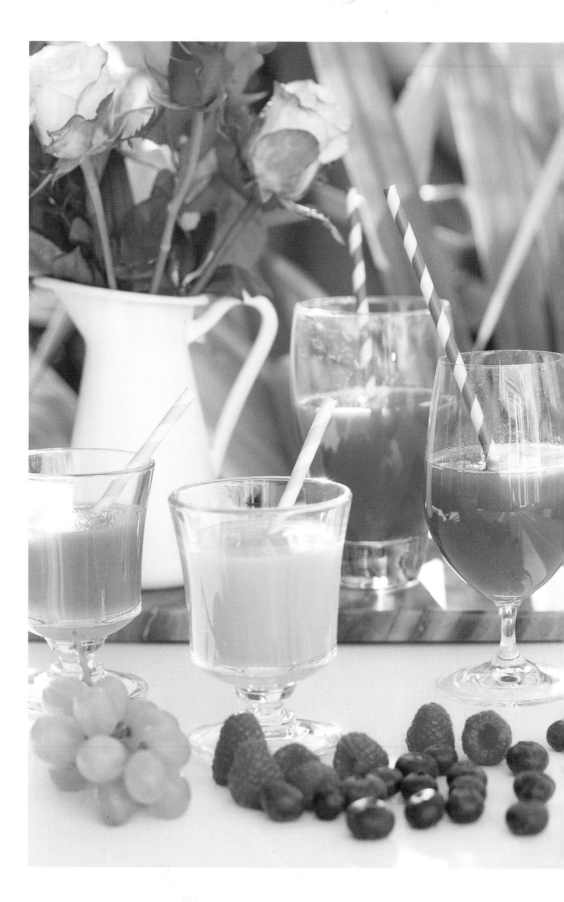

Beat the Bloat Juice
Serves 1

Fennel is great for aiding digestion.

Put all the ingredients into a blender. Top it up to the max with coconut water, some ice and blend.

Calories: Pineapple 93kcal

| 23g carbs | 4g fibre | 4g protein |

Calories: Apple 136kcal

| 38g carbs | 7g fibre | 3g protein |

100g cucumber

1 slice pineapple (or use an apple, peeled and cored)

¼ tsp fennel seeds

coconut water

ice

Morning Energiser
Serves 1

Put all the ingredients into a blender. Top it up to the max with water or unsweetened apple juice, some ice and blend.

Calories: 189kcal

| 47g carbs | 10g fibre | 1g protein | 1g fat |

1 apple

juice and zest of a lime

handful of blueberries or blackberries

10g oats

1 tsp chia seeds

½ tsp each of turmeric and cinnamon

water or apple juice (unsweetened)

ice

Post-Workout Smoothie
Serves 1

Put all the ingredients into a blender. Top up with ice and blend everything together until smooth and frothy.

Calories: 160kcal

9.5g carbs   3g fibre   24g protein   2.5g fat

200ml coconut water

zest and juice of half a lime

1 scoop of protein powder (I like the coconut and lime flavour but vanilla will work too. You should use your choice of whey or hemp protein if you are vegetarian)

ice

Growing Years Sneaky Smoothie
(Reproduced with kind permission of Glenisk)
Serves 2

This is a great one for kids – it nicely hides the spinach!

Tip everything into the blender and blend until smooth. Serve over ice.

Calories: 91kcal

16g carbs   2.4g fibre   1.5g protein   2g fat

125ml water

125ml fresh orange juice

80g strawberries

75g blueberries

30g spinach (or more if you can get it in!)

1 small Glenisk organic vanilla yoghurt.

ice

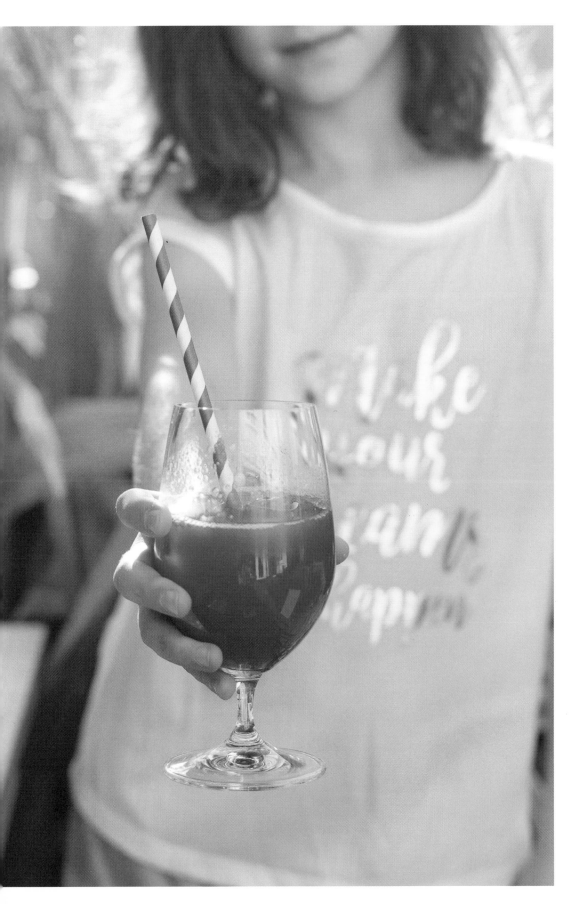

Beetroot and Orange Zinger
Serves 2

Tip everything into the blender and top up with water and ice.

Calories: 104kcal

23g carbs   1g fibre   3g protein

1 small cooked beetroot, chopped up

juice of 4 oranges, or blood oranges if in season

small knob of fresh ginger peeled and chopped

ice

Breakfast On The Run
Serves 1

When you have a busy day, and need breakfast quickly, the perfect smoothie for 1 is the answer.

Start with 1 scoop of protein powder and one large mug of your liquid of choice (milk, nut milk, coconut water, unsweetened apple juice, cold green tea)

Add ½ cup of frozen fruit and as many handfuls of green veg (spinach, kale, cucumber, fennel) as you can manage.

Throw in some boosters such as a handful of oats, hemp, chia or flax.

Add some spice if you fancy it, such as cinnamon, mixed spice, turmeric, ginger, lime or lemon zest.

Blend with loads of ice and there you have it!

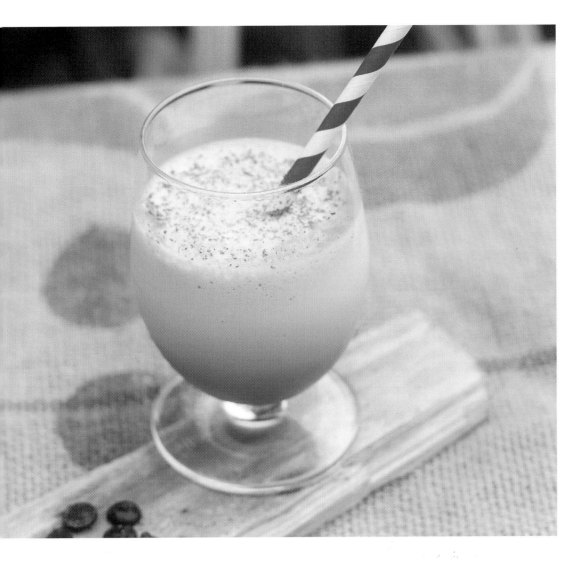

Cold-Brew Coffee Mocha
Serves 2

Perfect if you like coffee but are not inclined to eat breakfast. Great before a workout.

Brew your coffee in a French press (plunger) with cold water, ideally the night before and leave in the fridge overnight.

Put the coffee and protein powder into the blender and blend until smooth. Pour over ice and serve and top with a pinch of cinnamon.

400ml cold-brew coffee

2 scoops chocolate protein powder

ice

Calories: 119kcal

1.5g carbs   1g fibre   22g protein   2.5g fat

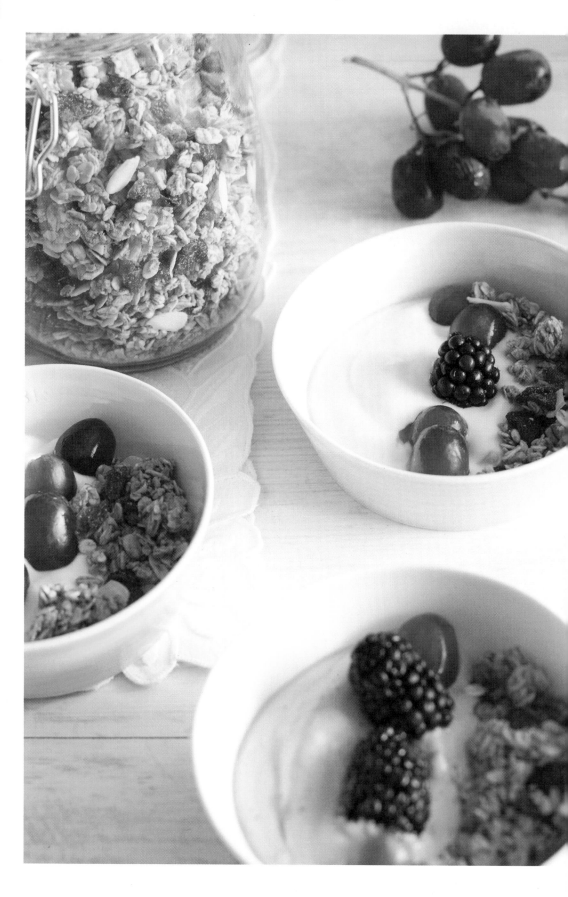

Homemade Granola
Makes 17 portions approx.

I love granola but tend to make it at home as the shop-bought varieties can be very sweet. Watch portion size – if you weigh out a serving of granola, you will see what a small amount it is yet the calories are high. I aim to use granola as a garnish – top some protein-loaded natural yoghurt with it and a few berries for a decent breakfast with a good nutritional balance of carbs, protein and fat. For a little sweet snack during the day, top a small yoghurt with a spoon of this. You don't need to be exact with the combining ingredients – a selection of nuts and dried fruit in similar ratios will work just as well.

Preheat oven to 170°C.

Melt the honey and oil together gently.

Combine the oats, barley flakes, rye flakes and pumpkin seeds. Add in the melted honey oil mix and stir well to combine.

Spread out on a roasting tray and bake for 20 minutes until golden brown. Stir the mixture after ten minutes to prevent uneven browning.

Allow to cool and combine with the wheatgerm, fruit, coconut flakes and nuts.

Store in an airtight tin or ziplock bag. It will keep for several weeks.

Serve a small portion with your favourite yoghurt and fruit for a delicious start to the day.

4 tbsp honey

100 ml light flavourless oil, or coconut oil if you like it

325g oats

100g barley flakes

50g rye flakes

25g pumpkin seeds

30g wheatgerm

100g dried fruit

25g coconut flakes

40g toasted hazelnuts

Calories per 40g portion
(Granola): 203kcal

25g carbs	3g fibre
4g protein	9.5g fat

Breakfast Flapjacks
Makes 24

When I first met Dominic, he was making these as a handy snack-cum-meal for when he was very busy with clients and not always able to take a proper break. He used to combine this with a protein shake, but I mostly have one with a fruit yoghurt – I like to buy the ones with added protein. This recipe makes a big batch of 24 which lasts us the week so feel free to halve the quantities. While these have none of the extra sugar of conventional flapjacks, calories are high so make sure not to eat too many at once.

Preheat oven to 180°C.

Melt the butter and honey together over a *gentle* heat.

Mix the oats with the dried fruit, spice and add a pinch of salt. Make a well in the middle, add the melted butter/honey mix and the water, and mix together until all the oats are incorporated. If it is a bit dry, just add some more water until it is all mixed in.

Tip into a large flat baking tray (38cm by 26cm) that has a 2cm lip all round. With damped hands, press the mixture firmly flat, pressing into all the corners.

Bake for around 20 minutes until golden brown. Rotate the tray after about ten minutes.

Let cool for about ten minutes before cutting into 24 portions. A pizza wheel is super for doing the job quickly. Let cool completely before removing.

750g porridge oats

300g butter

250g honey

350ml water

500g dried fruit of choice

1 tsp each of mixed spice and ginger

(optional extras include lemon or orange zest and some seeds if you like such as flax, pumpkin, poppy or sunflower seeds – a couple of handfuls total)

Calories: 301kcal

41g carbs	3.5g fibre
4.5g protein	12g fat

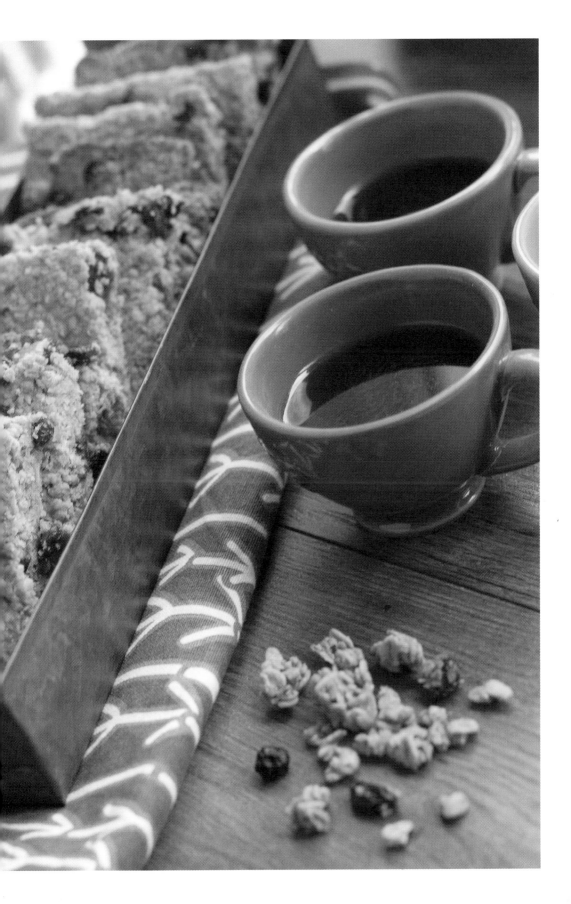

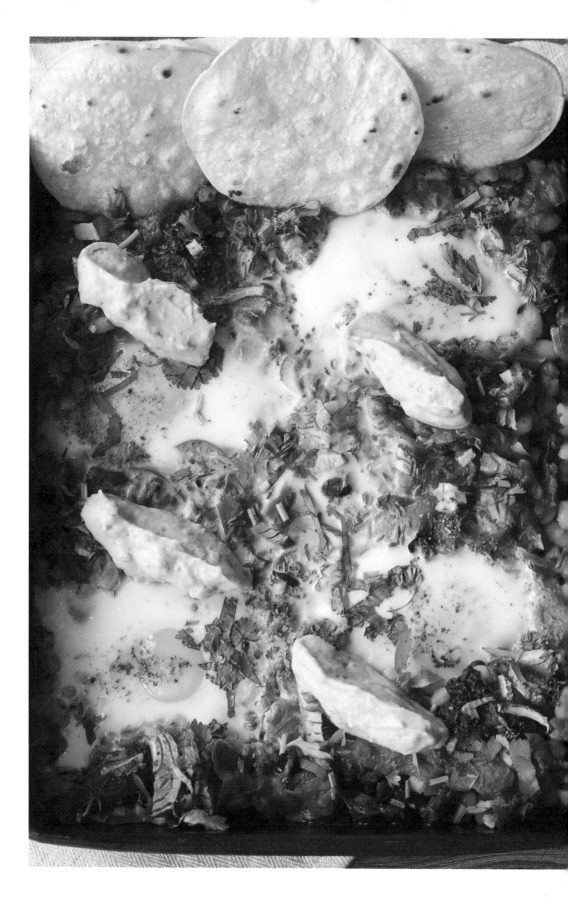

Huevos Rancheros
Serves 4

I was introduced to this on my J1 when I worked as a breakfast waitress on the Maryland shore in the late 1980s. I had never seen such enormous pancakes and waffles. Eggs are still my favourite breakfast food and this is my take on a classic spicy breakfast but without the deep-fried nachos.

Preheat oven to 180°C.

Put the beans into an ovenproof dish big enough to hold them in a single layer. Mix the chipotle with the tomatoes and pour over the beans. Sprinkle the red onion, cumin seeds and the oregano on top.

Make four wells and crack in the eggs.

Bake in the oven for about 15–20 minutes.

Sprinkle the coriander on top, with a spoon of guacamole on each egg.

Meanwhile toast the tortillas on a dry pan and serve 1 per egg.

2 tins black beans, rinsed and drained (net weight 480g)

1 x 400g tin tomatoes – drain some of the juice off

1 tsp chipotle in adobo

½ red onion, diced

1 tsp cumin seeds

1 tsp dried oregano or epazote if you can get it

4 eggs

2 tbsp fresh coriander, chopped

4 tbsp guacamole to serve (good quality from the chill section)

4 small tortillas/tostadas or slices of sourdough, toasted, to serve

Calories: 175kcal

| 12g carbs | 6g fibre | 12g protein | 11g fat |

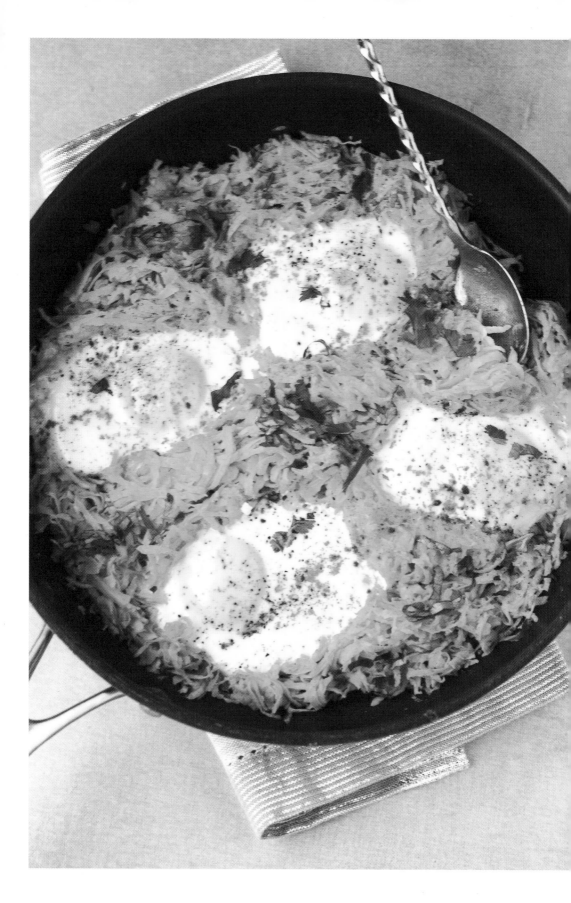

Sweet Potato Eggs
Serves 4

This is the most amazing dish, filling nutritious and so easy. You could make a few pans of this if you are having people over for brunch at the weekend. It makes a really tasty and easy meal when time is short midweek.

Tip the sweet potato into a bowl. Add the parsley and paprika and season to taste. Melt the butter in a large frying pan and tip all the sweet potato in. Stir to ensure it is well covered in the melted butter and then cook on a low/medium heat, stirring from time to time with a wooden spoon. The sweet potato will be almost cooked after about ten minutes.

Make four wells and add the eggs. Cover the pan with a lid or large plate, turn the heat down to low/medium and cook the eggs to your liking. They will cook gently rather than fry and are lovely!

As an alternative, you could finish in the oven at 180°C – it takes about ten minutes for the egg white to set.

1 large sweet potato, peeled and grated

4 tbsp flat-leaf parsley, chopped

1 tsp sweet paprika

25g butter

4 eggs

Calories: 230kcal

25g carbs   4g fibre   8.5g protein   11g fat

Breakfast Mini Omelettes
Makes 12

These are very handy for breakfast and lunch. I use frozen vegetables – red peppers and mixed greens – for my fillings but there are many variations you can try.

Preheat oven to 170°C.

Grease a 12-cup muffin tin.

Chop the pancetta and add to a bowl.

Heat the oil and add the onion. Cook until soft and translucent.

Add to bowl with pancetta. Add the peppers and thyme to the pan, season and cook until soft. Tip into the bowl, take out the thyme, and set aside. Divide the filling into the muffin cups.

Beat the eggs in the milk and pour into the muffin cups. Put into the oven for 12–15 minutes until puffed up and cooked through. Remove from the oven and let cool slightly before removing from the tin.

75g pancetta or ham of choice

1 tbsp oil

1 small onion, finely chopped

150g chopped peppers

1 sprig of thyme

5 eggs, beaten

100ml milk

Calories: 64kcal

1.5g carbs	trace fibre	5g protein	4g fat

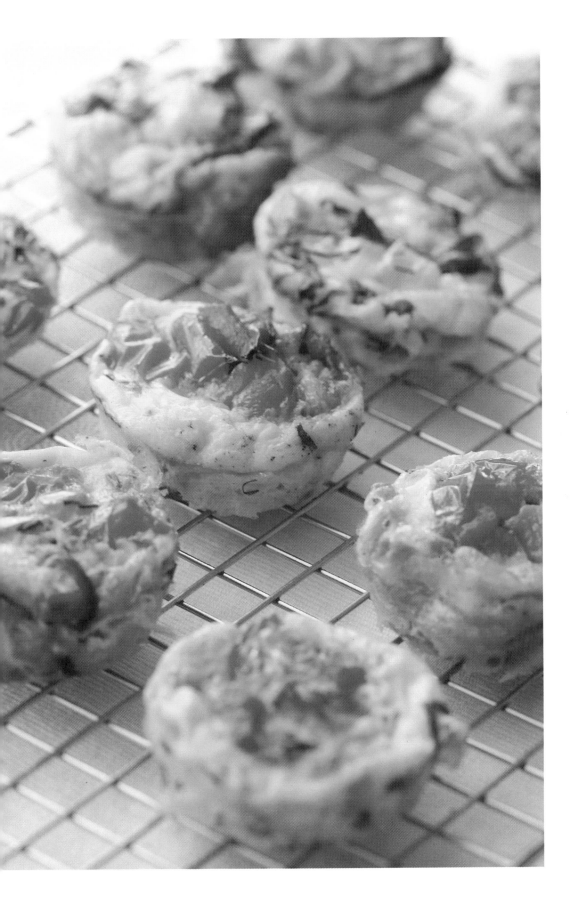

Bean Frittata
Serves 3

This is great for a hearty breakfast or lunch. Eggs are versatile – easy to cook with and so nutritious! – and the beans make it that bit more filling. You could us any canned cooked beans you like (not the sweet ones in sauce, though!). If I am making this for all the family, I tend to leave out the chilli.

Break eggs into a bowl and beat well.

Add in chilli, garlic, pepper and beans. Gently stir in the chopped herbs.

Melt the oil in a frying pan.

Tip mixture into the pan and cook on low heat for about ten minutes. From time to time, lift the edge to allow more mixture to flow in to cook. Finish under the grill or, using a plate, gently flip the frittata over and cook on the other side until cooked through. Ensure there is no runny egg or you will burn yourself. It should be cooked through in about five minutes.

Cut into wedges and serve.

6 eggs

1 red chilli, deseeded and chopped

1 clove of garlic, peeled, mashed and chopped

1 small cooked red pepper, chopped

1 can of cannellini beans, rinsed and drained (240g drained weight)

2 tbsp each of flat-leaf parsley and chives, chopped

1 tbsp oil

Calories: 262kcal

13.5g carbs   6g fibre   18g protein   14g fat

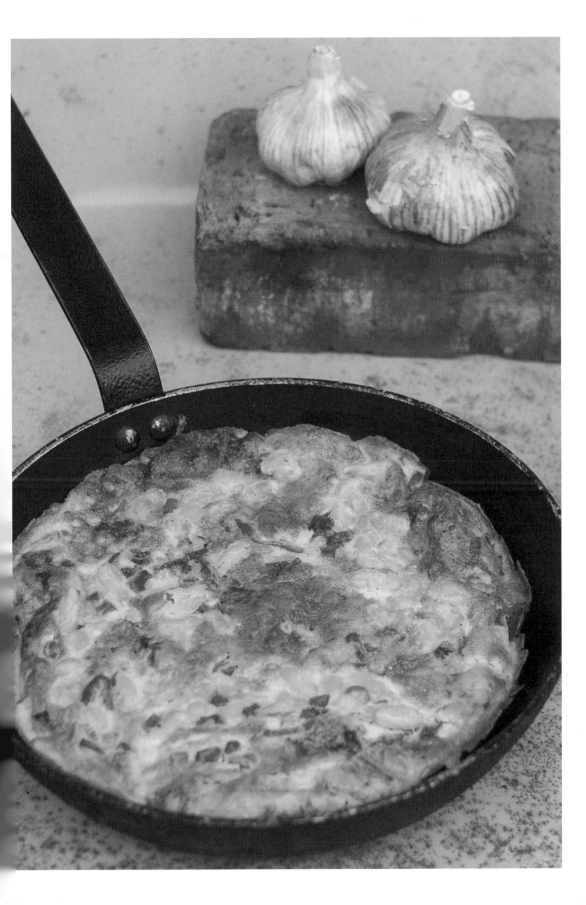

Scrambled Eggs with Peppers and Spinach
Serves 2

I use frozen spinach and peppers regularly as they are handy to keep in the freezer. When I plan to make this, I just take out what I need the night before or if I have forgotten to, I simply stick the spinach and peppers in a colander and run some cool water over them to help them defrost quickly.

Heat the oil, add peppers and fry gently until softening.

Add the spinach and cook gently for about five minutes until both are soft. If a lot of water has been released from the spinach, drain this off before adding the eggs.

Stir in the eggs, sprinkle with the paprika, and cook over a medium heat. Make sure to stir from time to time, to scramble.

Cook for about 3 minutes or until set.

½ tbsp rapeseed oil

100g chopped, frozen peppers

100g frozen spinach, defrosted and drained

4 large eggs, lightly beaten

1 tsp paprika

Calories: 190kcal

4g carbs   2g fibre   14g protein   12.5g fat

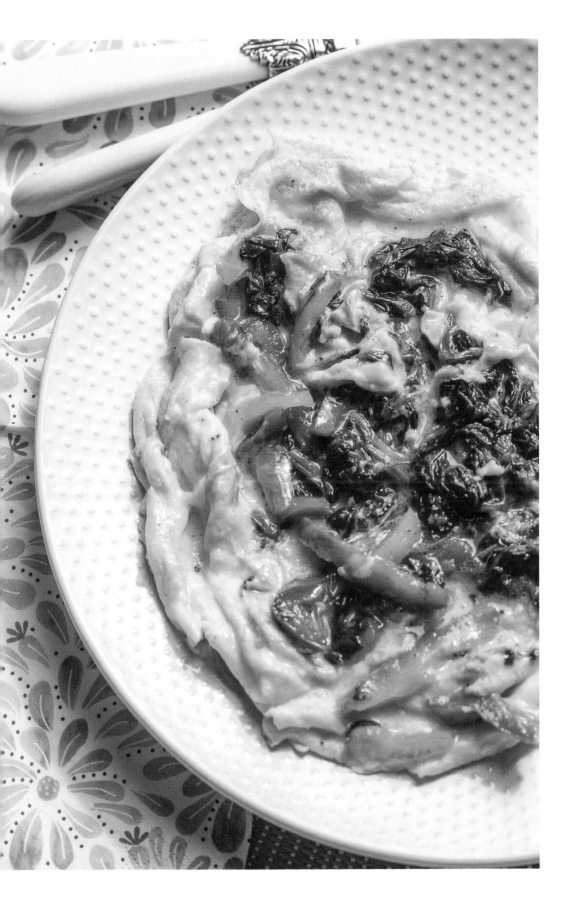

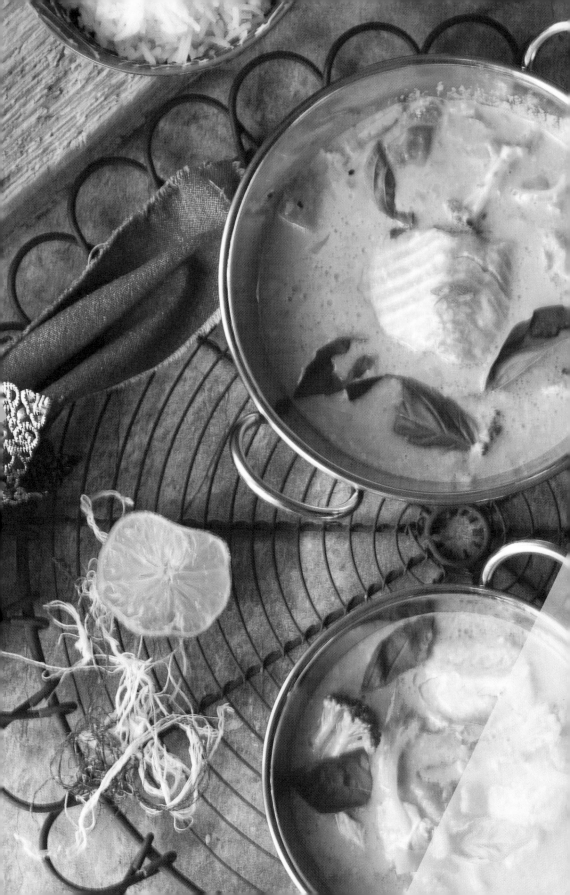

Mains

We eat meat but much less than in the past, probably less than once a week, hence these recipes have a fish, poultry and plant slant. In the last ten years, we consciously upped the number of times a week we have a plant-based dinner and love how we feel on this kind of food, as well as the impact it has had on our family food budget. All the Bluezones research (places in the world which have populations that live healthier and longer lives) and analysis show that a plant slant in your diet is a contributor to health and longevity. The thing to remember is to make a complete plant-based protein by combining grains and nuts, legumes and seeds or grains or nuts.

Eating in front of the TV is a distraction to precious time together as well as to our digestion.

Handy tips

Oils

This is an area to watch out for. I love oils and the body needs good fats but I try to add them in the form of dressings and marinades where I can be aware of the portion rather than chucking loads into a pot when I need to cook off veg or meat for a recipe. A tablespoon of any oil contains approximately 9g of fat and close to 90 calories so you can see how easy it could be to overdo it. There are issues with overheating oils so I never heat the oils hot and usually add a tablespoon or two of water to the oil when I am cooking off veg at the start of a recipe. If I am cooking off meat or fish, I use a cooking spray as it is easy to control how much is used.

Lemon or lime juice

My favourite flavour enhancer! I add a squeeze of lemon or lime juice or some zest to many dishes, both sweet and savoury, to enhance the flavours in the food. Add just before serving and taste the results to see how much difference it makes. You could also try a drizzle of your favourite vinegar.

Preparing veg ahead of time

I blanch or steam a lot of vegetables until they are almost fully cooked. They will sit happily in the fridge until needed and are ready very quickly when you are prepping a midweek dinner. This will work for broccoli, carrots, beans, etc., and is a great time-saving trick.

Fresh herbs and spices

Get as many fresh herbs and spices as you can into your cooking. They contain phytonutrients, essential oils, vitamins and minerals, albeit in small quantities, are still believed to help reduce inflammation in the body, some have antibacterial properties, can improve digestion, help upset stomachs, sooth sore throats, as well as adding amazing flavour to your food. I always have fresh mint, coriander, parsley and chives in the fridge. Rosemary and thyme can be grown easily in the garden or in a window pot. I have loads of spices in my press and they never get too old as I use them so regularly. The ones I use most often are chilli, cumin, coriander, nigella seeds, turmeric, paprika, cayenne, and I always have ginger and garlic to hand. I find the jars of chopped chillis under oil, cooked red peppers and garlic puree great to have in the press.

The freezer is your lifesaver	Batch cook and freeze the surplus. This is great for midweek meals. Instead of having to start from scratch when you are tired after a day at work, you can take the food out in the morning and it is ready to reheat when you are home. I use strong freezer bags and flatten the portions to make them much easier to store and to defrost (especially if like us, you don't have a microwave).
Beans	We have a plant slant in our diet and eat loads of beans in the form of casseroles, burgers, dips and salads. They are a good source of protein, and great for adding fibre into your diet and helping you feel full, as well as aiding your digestion, due to the fibre. However, they are high in FODMAPs so if you have a gut disorder, you may find that they trigger your symptoms. If you haven't eaten many before, you may find they affect you in other ways but that should settle down.
Handy Ingredients	Jars of cooked peppers Good-quality yellow and red curry paste Miso paste Jars of mashed chillies in oil Frozen mixed fruit Frozen spinach, peas, mixed peppers and beans (I don't like frozen broccoli or cauliflower as they are very watery when they defrost).
Suppliers	I use some more slightly unusual ingredients such as ancho chillies, epazote and chipotle in adobo. If you are in Ireland I highly recommend www.PicadoMexican.com, an online Mexican ingredient website that will deliver to your door and, for your Asian staples, www.asiamarket.ie.

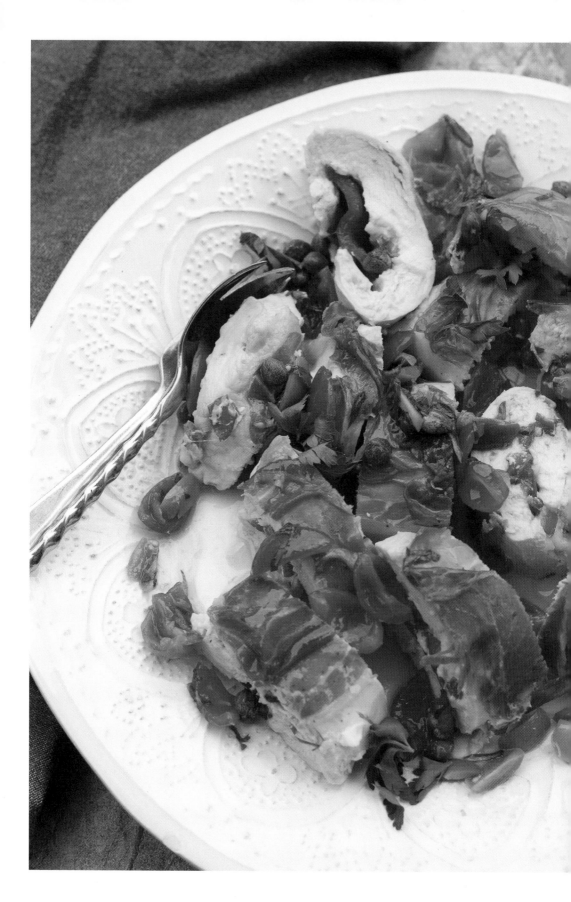

Sicilian-style Stuffed Chicken Breasts with Caper and Olive Dressing
Serves 4

With olives, chillis and capers, this is a real taste of Sicily and is one of my favourite chicken dishes. It is also good for bringing to work the next day, with a big leafy salad.

Preheat the oven to 180°C.

Place the chicken on a piece of cling film, cover with more cling film and bash flat. Lay the ham down on chopping board and top with the chicken breast.

Spread a teaspoon of the chillis over the chicken, top with the mozzarella and the pepper. Tightly roll up so that it is a bit like a Swiss roll. Spray the base of an ovenproof casserole with one spray of oil.

Place the chicken in the dish, season and cook for approximately 20 minutes.

Serve sliced, with caper and olive dressing drizzled over.

For the dressing

Combine all the ingredients in a small bowl and pour over the chicken.

4 medium chicken breasts

4 slices Parma ham

4 tsp chopped chilli peppers

1 small mozzarella ball, cut into 8 slices

1 medium cooked red pepper (from a jar) sliced in 4

salt and pepper

Dressing

2 tsp capers, drained

4 green olives, deseeded and sliced

4 cherry tomatoes, deseeded and chopped

handful of fresh parsley, chopped

40ml olive oil

Juice of half a lemon

Calories: Sicilian-style stuffed Chicken Breasts 210kcal

2.5g carbs   33g protein   7.5g fat

Calories: Dressing 100kcal

2.5g carbs   10g fat

Total: 310kcal

5g carbs   33g protein   17.5g fat

Serving Suggestion: Serve with the sumac carrots or roast baby potatoes.

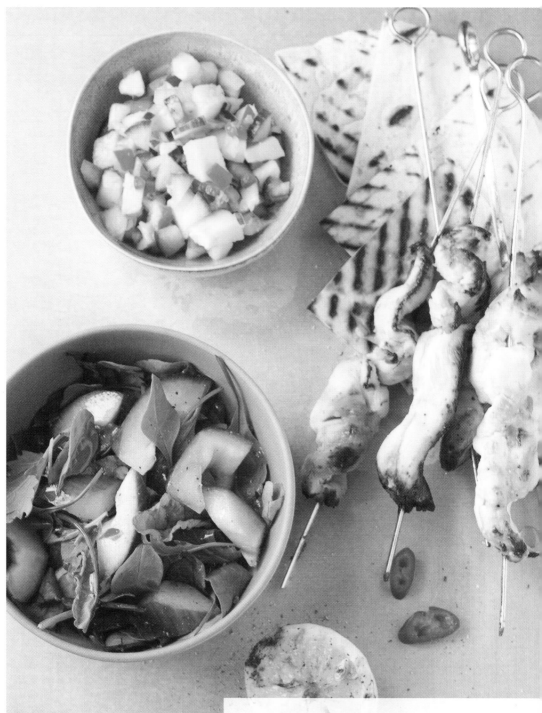

Calories: 241kcal

28g carbs   3g fibre   27g protein   4g fat

Add a wrap: 94kcal

18g carbs   2g fat

Sweet Chilli and Lime Chicken with Mango Salsa
Serves 4

This is a delicious way to serve chicken, rich in vitamins, minerals and antioxidant compounds. No ketchup or mustard required here: just spoon on the salsa and eat. This keeps well so double up and bring some for lunch the next day. Serve in a wrap for an extra 100kcals.

Cut each chicken breast into four lengths.

Tip into a bowl with all the marinade ingredients and toss well to combine. Leave to marinate for 30 minutes or, if you can, a few hours in the fridge, covered.

Thread onto the skewers if you are using – 2 pieces per skewer. Cover the handles with a little tinfoil if they are wooden.

Heat a griddle pan (or you can grill them – just adjust the cooking time to about four or five minutes a side). Cook the chicken thoroughly – about three minutes per side in the griddle pan.

Tip the rest of the marinade into a pot, bring to the boil. Boil for two minutes then reduce and gently simmer until slightly thicker. Pour into a serving bowl and set aside. (It is safe to do this with the marinade as long as you bring it to the boil and cook as instructed.)

Make the mango salsa by combining everything and leaving to stand for a few minutes for flavours to develop.

Combine the salad greens and cucumber slices. Serve the chicken with the mango salsa and the green salad, drizzle with the marinade and lastly a squeeze of lime juice.

4 chicken breasts off the bone

8 skewers (soak if wooden)
Optional

Marinade

finely grated zest and juice of a lime

2 tbsp soy sauce, tamari (gluten-free soy) or coconut aminos (try your local health store. They are are from the sap of the coconut tree and add a lovely flavour - similar but better in my opinion than soy)

2.5cm piece of ginger peeled and grated

1 tbsp honey

½ tsp salt

½ red chilli, deseeded and very finely chopped

1 clove garlic, mashed

salt and pepper to season

Salsa

2 mangos, peeled and diced

1 small red onion, diced very finely

½ red pepper, diced very finely

juice and zest of 1 lime

1 tbsp chopped coriander

1 tbsp olive oil

Green Salad

4 handfuls of mixed salad leaves

¼ cucumber, deseeded and sliced

Chicken Breasts with Honey and Lemon
Serves 4

The marinade in this recipe is simple and easy but so delicious, a taste of summer on the plate!

Preheat oven to 180°C.

Add all ingredients together bar the chicken and whisk to combine.

Dry the chicken breasts thoroughly and place in a roasting tin.

Pour half the marinade over the chicken breasts, taking care to cover them well.

Roast in the oven for 40 minutes approximately, until cooked through and juices run clear. Halfway through cooking, baste the chicken breasts with the rest of the marinade and continue cooking until they are lovely and golden and fully cooked.

juice of 1 lemon

50ml honey

1 tbsp fresh thyme, chopped finely

1 tbsp rosemary, chopped finely

1 clove garlic, finely mashed

4 medium chicken breasts on the bone

Serving Suggestion:
Serve with green beans, mangetout or carrots and a portion of butter bean or chickpea mash.

Calories: 230kcal

9g carbs   30g protein   8g fat

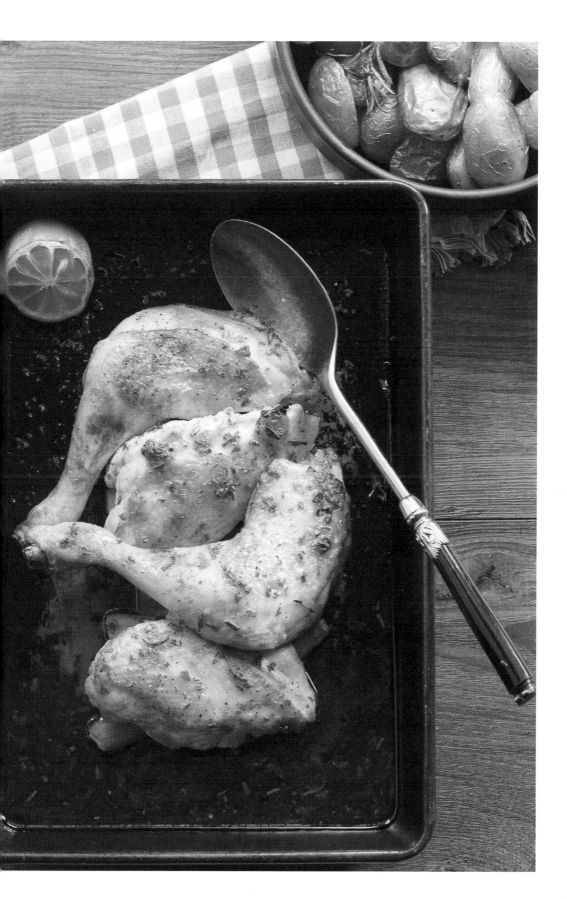

Chicken and Vegetable Bake
Serves 6

This is a complete meal with nothing else needed. A rich treat and a real family pleaser in our house, the parmesan and cream are filling. If you don't like cream you could use a tin of coconut milk instead. You could do this with a whole chicken poached, also.

Preheat oven to 180°C.

Poach the chicken in the stock on a gentle heat until just cooked. Fork apart and tip into a casserole dish and set aside.

Add shallot, garlic and herbes de Provence to a pan with a spray of oil and cook for a minute or two until softening. Add some water if needed. Add the cream and stock, mix and season.

Add the sweet potato slices into the liquid and cook for about five minutes until softening.

Spoon this over the chicken in the baking dish. Arrange the slices to cover the chicken, then top with the cauliflower and sprinkle with the cheese.

Bake for about 20 minutes until golden brown and cooked through.

6 medium chicken breasts

200ml chicken or vegetable stock – feel free to use a bought stock or stock mix

1 medium shallot, peeled and finely chopped

2 cloves garlic, finely mashed

1 heaped tsp herbes de Provence

100ml pouring cream

1 large sweet potato, peeled and thinly sliced

1 medium head of cauliflower, trimmed and thinly sliced

50g grated Parmesan

Calories: 298kcal

| 22g carbs | 4g fibre | 31.5 protein | 10g fat |

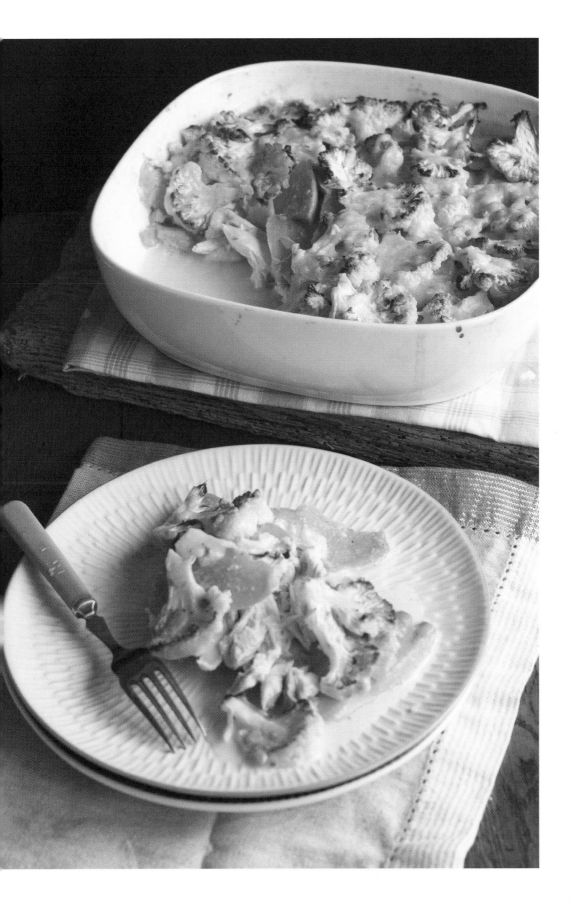

Marinated Spicy Chicken with Cauliflower Puree
Serves 6

This chicken recipe is perfect if you want to cook extra and have it for lunch at work or school.

For the chicken
Combine the marinade ingredients and toss the chicken in and marinate, covered in the fridge for a couple of hours, or overnight if you can. Heat a heavy-bottomed pan or griddle, remove the chicken from the marinade and cook on the pan for about five minutes per side until cooked through. Remove and keep warm.

For the cauliflower
Trim the cauliflower into florets and tip into a wide pan. Barely cover with the water/milk mixture. Add the bay leaf. Bring to the boil, reduce to a simmer and cook for about 20 minutes until tender. Reserve the liquid and tip the cauliflower into a blender with the bay leaf, olive oil and blend until smooth. Add the liquid as needed until you have a lovely smooth, silky puree. Taste and season if needed. Keep warm while you plate up.

Spoon some cauliflower puree onto a plate and serve with a chicken breast.

Chicken Marinade

100ml olive oil

4 garlic cloves, mashed

2 bay leaves

1 tbsp sweet paprika

1 tbsp oregano

1 tsp fennel seeds, pounded

1 tsp ground cumin

6 chicken fillets, off the bone and flattened

Cauliflower Puree

1 large cauliflower

Water/milk to cover (about 100ml milk topped up with 150ml water)

1 bay leaf

10ml olive oil

Calories: 220kcal

10g carbs   3.5g fibre   28.5 protein   8g fat

Serving Suggestion: Lovely with the green beans or carrots.

I have experimented several times with the marinades and approximately 30 per cent of a marinade stays on the chicken and the rest is discarded.

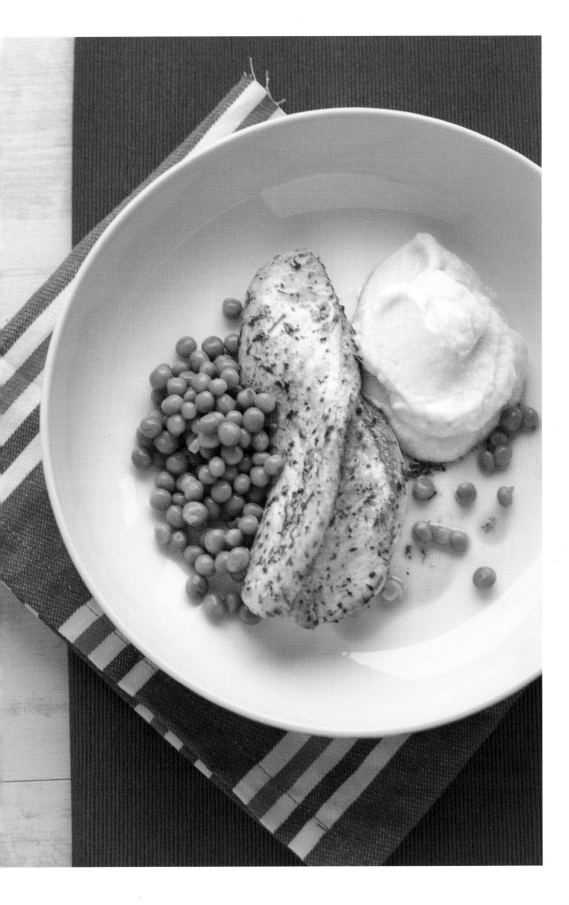

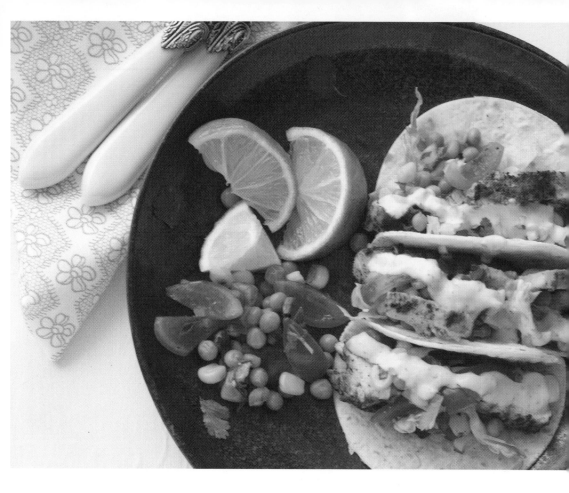

Spicy Chicken Tostadas, Colourful Mixed Salad and Ranch-style Dressing
Serves 6

For the Chicken

Combine all the marinade ingredients, toss the chicken in and marinate, covered in the fridge for a couple of hours or overnight if you have time. Heat a heavy bottomed pan or griddle, remove the chicken from the marinade and cook it on the pan for about five minutes per side until cooked through. Remove, slice and keep warm.

For the chicken

100ml olive oil

1 tsp fennel seeds, lightly crushed

4 garlic cloves, mashed

1 tbsp sweet paprika

1 tbsp epazote or oregano

1 tsp ground cumin

2 bay leaves

6 chicken fillets, off the bone and flattened

Mixed Vegetable Salad

200g cherry tomatoes, cut in half

200g cooked peas

25g cooked corn

4 tbsp chopped coriander

1 small red or white onion, very finely sliced

juice and zest of ½ lime

For the Mixed Vegetable Salad

Combine everything and set aside until needed.

For the Ranch-style Dressing

Combine everything except the coriander. Taste and season as needed. Just before serving, add the coriander and stir gently.

To serve

Warm the tortillas/tostadas on a dry pan for about one minute per side.

Pile some salad leaves on top. Spoon over the vegetable salad. Top with some sliced chicken and drizzle over the spicy dressing.

Ranch-style Dressing

1 tbsp mayonnaise

4 tbsp Greek-style natural yoghurt

2 tsp buttermilk – If you don't have this handy you can replace with milk and a tiny squeeze of lemon juice.

juice of 1 lime

1 tsp brown sugar

1 tsp chipotle in adobo

1 clove garlic, finely mashed

½ tsp sweet paprika

a pinch each of dried thyme, oregano and fennel, or a large pinch of epazote if you have it

4 tbsp chopped fresh coriander

To finish

100g chopped lettuce or mixed leaves

2–3 mini tortillas/tostadas per person (or 1 wrap, if preferred)

Calories: 334kcal

33g carbs   2g fibre   27.5g protein   10g fat

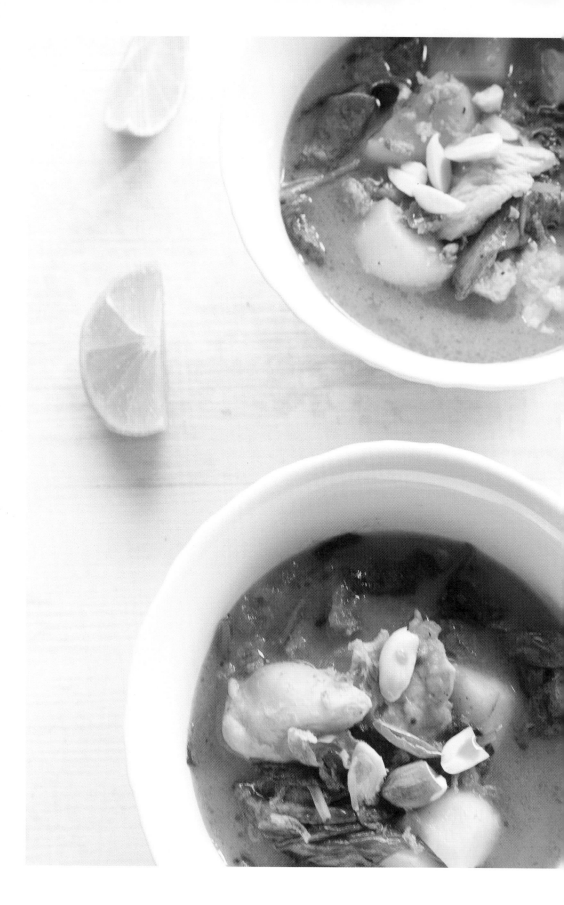

Quick Thai-style Midweek Chicken Curry
Serves 4–5

Using a good-quality shop-bought curry paste turns any dish into a quick weeknight favourite. I buy curry paste from the Asia Market in Dublin city centre, which is one of my favourite shops ever, even if purely for the theatre of watching the world go by. This recipe could be even quicker if you have any leftover cooked chicken, which could simply be tossed into the sauce.

Heat the oil, add the onion and cook until soft and tender (about five minutes).

Add the curry paste and stir well. Cook out until fragrant. This will take about three minutes.

Add the potatoes, chicken, coconut milk and water, and bring to a boil. Reduce the heat to a very gentle simmer. Cook, stirring occasionally, until the chicken is cooked, the potatoes are tender and there is a lovely oil shimmer on the top from the paste.

Just before serving, stir in the fish sauce, soy sauce and palm sugar, and then stir in the spinach and the lime juice. This makes four large or five medium servings.

Serve over rice. For those who like theirs hotter, simply thinly slice a red chilli and toss over the served dish.

1 tbsp oil

1 small onion, sliced thinly

1 heaped tbsp yellow curry paste

1lb potatoes, peeled and cut into 1cm pieces

1lb skinless boneless chicken pieces (around 2.5cm each)

1 400ml tin light coconut milk

400ml water

1 tbsp fish sauce

1 tbsp tamari or coconut aminos or soy sauce if you don't have either

1 tsp palm sugar to season

4 large handfuls spinach

1 tbsp lime juice

Rice, to serve

Calories: 285kcal

| 26g carbs | 3g fibre | 26g protein | 8.5g fat |

With rice
Total Calories: 385kcal

| 49g carbs | 5g fibre | 29g protein | 9.5g fat |

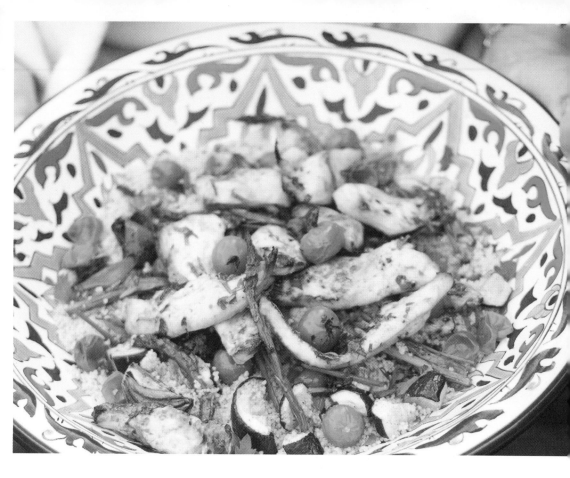

Spicy Chicken with Roasted Vegetables, Sumac Couscous and Herb Dressing
Serves 4

This can also be made with prawns. They will cook quickly under the grill – just three minutes a side until done. Remember to soak your skewers if using wooden ones! The herb dressing really lifts this dish and adds loads of extra flavour.

For the Roasted Vegetables

Put all the ingredients into a bowl, season, then spray with oil and mix well. Tip onto a baking tray and roast at 170°C for about 15 minutes until tender and cooked. Set aside.

Roasted Vegetables

1 medium courgette, diced

1 medium red onion, sliced

150g cherry tomatoes, halved

100g asparagus, trimmed as needed

2 sprays of oil

½ tsp salt

Chicken

4 chicken breasts, cut into strips

2 tbsp honey

1 clove of garlic, finely mashed

half a red chilli, finely chopped or 1 tsp mashed chillies under oil

1 tbsp oil

Sumac Couscous

1 tsp sumac (this is a berry which is dried and has a tangy lemon flavour. If you can't get this, substitute with 1 tsp lemon zest)

100g couscous, or quinoa if you prefer

110ml boiling water

Herb Dressing

3 tbsp chives, chopped

3 tbsp flat-leaf parsley, chopped

3 tbsp mint

2 tbsp olive oil

For the Chicken

Mix all the ingredients and marinate the chicken for at least 30 minutes in the fridge.

Grill the chicken for about four minutes a side until cooked through and nicely golden.

For the Sumac Couscous

Tip couscous into bowl. Add the sumac and stir. Cover with the water and set aside for about ten minutes. If you are replacing with quinoa, add the sumac to the dry quinoa and follow the cooking instructions on the pack.

Fluff up with a fork and cool until needed.

For the Herb Dressing

Set aside one third of the herbs for the top and combine the rest in the olive oil.

To assemble

Tip the couscous/quinoa into a bowl, mix in the roasted veg and season well. Add the chicken on the top, sprinkle on the extra chopped herbs and drizzle over the herb dressing.

Calories: 350kcal

| 34g carbs | 2.5g fibre |
| 30g protein | 11.5g fat |

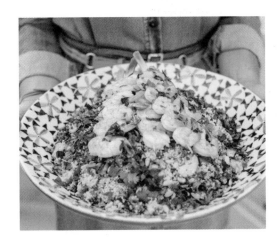

Turkey Meatballs in Masala Sauce
Serves 4

Turkey is a great lean protein and these meatballs are full of lovely flavour with a hint of heat. These would also be delicious with the spiced lentils recipe. Beware the turkey drying out – use a meat thermometer, if you have one.

For the meatballs

Put the turkey mince into a bowl, add all the other ingredients, mix well and shape into 16 meatballs. Cover with cling film and leave in the fridge for at least 30 minutes for the flavours to develop – the longer you wait, the better the flavour.

For the masala sauce

Heat the oil, add the onion and sweat for about two minutes until it softens. Add a splash of water if needed.

Add the ginger and garlic and cook for a further three minutes.

Stir in the spices then cook for a minute or two. Add a splash of water if it seems too dry.

Add the tomatoes and coconut milk and stir to combine. Bring to the boil briefly, then reduce to a gentle simmer and add the turkey meatballs.

Cook the meatballs in the sauce over a medium heat for about eight minutes, then turn them over and cook for about another eight minutes until cooked through. Splash the sauce over them occasionally to ensure they don't go dry. Just before serving, add the chopped kale and the squeeze of lime juice. Stir to combine and leave for a minute before serving. Serve over rice.

Meatballs

400g turkey mince –free range or organic is preferable

2 tbsp fresh coriander, chopped

2 tbsp mint, chopped

1 red chilli, chopped finely, or 1 tsp of chopped chilli in oil

1 tsp chopped fresh ginger

1 spring onion, peeled and chopped finely

1 tbsp fresh parsley, chopped

zest of a lime and juice of half

Masala sauce

½ tbsp rapeseed or coconut oil

1 medium white onion, finely diced

2cm piece fresh ginger, peeled and grated

2 cloves of garlic, finely mashed

1 tsp garam masala

1 tsp mild curry powder (if you like hotter, use it)

1 tsp turmeric

½ can chopped tomatoes (about 200g)

400ml tin of light coconut milk

80g kale, cleaned and finely chopped, or spinach if you prefer

a squeeze of lime juice

rice, to serve

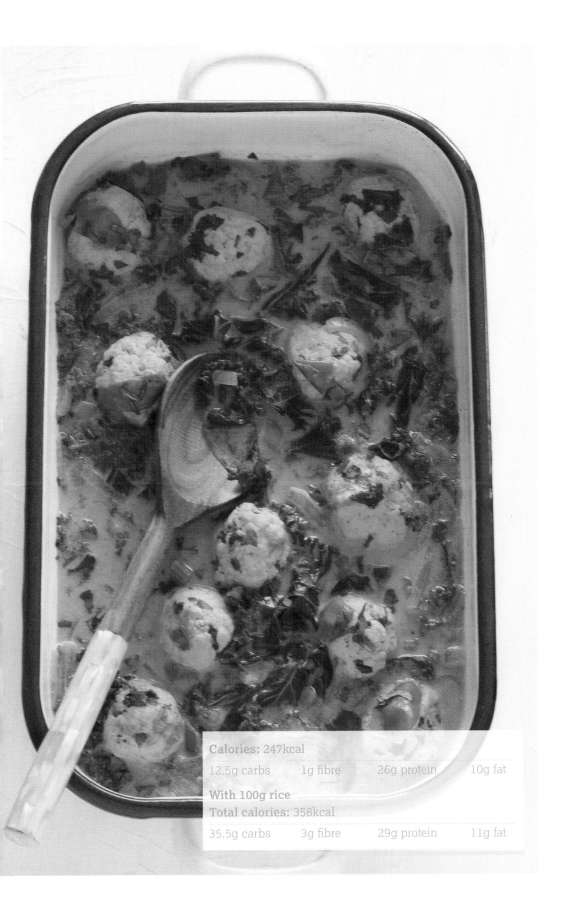

Calories: 247kcal

| 12.5g carbs | 1g fibre | 26g protein | 10g fat |

With 100g rice
Total calories: 358kcal

| 35.5g carbs | 3g fibre | 29g protein | 11g fat |

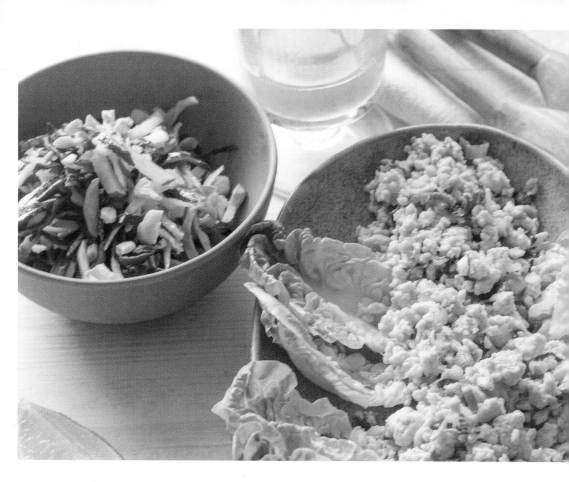

Turkey Lettuce Wraps with Asian Slaw
Serves 4

Heat the oil in a frying pan over a medium heat.

Add the onion, garlic, ginger and chilli and cook for about five minutes until softened. Put into a bowl while you cook the turkey.

Tip in the mince, season well with salt and pepper, if using, and cook, stirring until the turkey is almost cooked (about ten minutes). Add the onion mix back in.

Stir in the lime juice, fish sauce, aminos or tamari and let the flavours develop over a medium heat while it finishes cooking. Stir occasionally to make sure it doesn't catch.

½ tbsp rapeseed oil

1 small onion, finely chopped

2 cloves garlic, finely mashed

2.5cm piece of ginger, peeled and finely chopped

1 red chilli, deseeded and finely chopped

400g turkey mince

salt and pepper (if you use them)

juice and zest of 1 lime

2 tbsp fish sauce

1 tbsp liquid aminos or tamari (or soy sauce if you can't get these)

To finish

2 tbsp fresh mint, chopped

4 tbsp fresh coriander, chopped

3 spring onions, chopped

1 head of little gem lettuce,
separated into leaves and washed

Lime Dressing

zest of 1 lime and juice of 2

2 tbsp fish sauce

1 tsp palm sugar

Asian Slaw

100g red cabbage, finely shredded.

100g white cabbage, finely
shredded

2 spring onions, finely chopped

50g mangetout

50g sugar snaps

50g radish, finely chopped

1 tbsp rice wine vinegar

2 tbsp rapeseed oil

1 tsp sesame oil

1 tbsp liquid aminos or tamari (or
soy sauce, if you can't find these)

½–1 tsp chilli flakes, according to
taste

25g chopped cashews

Let it cool a little, then stir in the herbs and
spring onions and sprinkle the lime zest over.
Fill the lettuce leaves with the mixture and
top with the lime dressing and serve with the
Asian slaw.

For the Lime Dressing

Mix everything together and drizzle over the
filled lettuce leaves.

For the Asian Slaw

Toss all the vegetables together and season
well.

Make the dressing by whisking together rice
wine vinegar, rapeseed and sesame oil, aminos
and the chilli flakes.

Toss over the vegetables, combine very well
and sprinkle the cashews on top.

Slaw Calories: 129kcal

| 10g carbs | 2g fibre | 2.25g protein | 9g fat |

Total Calories: 297kcal

| 20g carbs | 3.25g fibre | 28g protein | 12g fat |

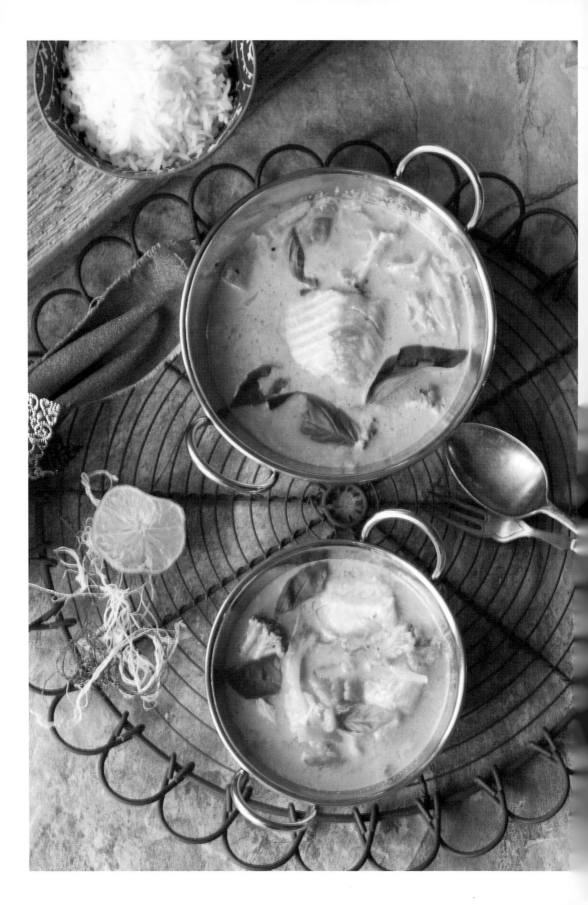

Salmon in a Coconut Turmeric Sauce
Serves 4

Salmon is nutritionally dense and something of a superfood but you can substitute it with any juicy thick fish fillets you like; indeed, you could throw in prawns instead (just adjust the cooking time down to about two or three minutes until the prawns are opaque). In this recipe, you are getting lots of good fat. It is really filling and needs nothing more than perhaps a side dish of one of the green vegetable recipes or rice if you would like to make it go further.

Heat the oil in a wide pan or pot, add the onion and sweat for about two minutes until it softens. Add the ginger, garlic and lemongrass and cook for another five minutes.

Stir in the spices and cook for a minute or two. Add a splash of water if it seems too dry.

Add the tomatoes, coconut milk and water, and stir to combine. Bring to a very gentle boil, then reduce to a low simmer and cook for about ten minutes to develop the flavour. Taste and add the palm sugar as needed. Stir, then add the salmon.

Cook the fish in the sauce over a gentle medium heat – splash the sauce over the fish occasionally. It should take about eight minutes to cook through. Stir in the chopped coriander or basil leaves, the lime juice and serve.

(You could also add in a few handfuls of spinach to the sauce, which would be equally delicious.)

½ tbsp rapeseed or coconut oil

1 medium white onion, finely sliced

2cm piece fresh ginger, peeled and grated

2 cloves of garlic, finely mashed

1 lemongrass (the bottom 2cm only only), peeled and finely chopped

1 tsp garam masala

1 tsp turmeric

1 400ml tin chopped tomatoes, drained of most of the juice

1 400ml tin of light coconut milk

150ml water

1 tsp palm sugar

4 medium salmon fillets

1 tbsp chopped fresh coriander to finish, or a few Thai basil leaves, if you can get them; if not, just use the coriander. (Thai Basil has a slightly aniseed flavour so don't substitute with regular basil.)

juice of ½ lime, to taste

Calories: 316kcal

9g carbs	1g fibre
21.5g protein	21g fat

Serving Suggestion:
Serve with one of the green veg or a side of rice

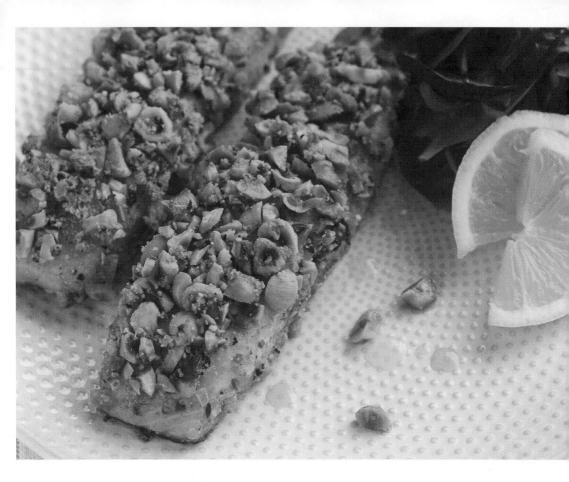

Harissa Salmon with Crunchy Nut Topping
Serves 4

Any nut you like can be substituted. This would be lovely with the spiced greens.

Preheat oven to 180°C.

Line an ovenproof dish with parchment.

Spread the nuts on a flat plate.

Coat each piece of salmon with some of the harissa paste, then press into the nuts to coat.

If you can, chill for about ten minutes.

Remove from the fridge, add about 50ml water to the dish (not on top of the salmon, just around it).

Bake for about ten minutes until cooked through.

85g cashew nuts and hazelnuts, finely chopped or blitzed (not pulverised)

4 salmon pieces

2 tsp harissa paste

Calories: 327kcal

| 6g carbs | 1.5g fibre |
| 23g protein | 23.75g fat |

Serving Suggestion:
Serve with the spiced greens.

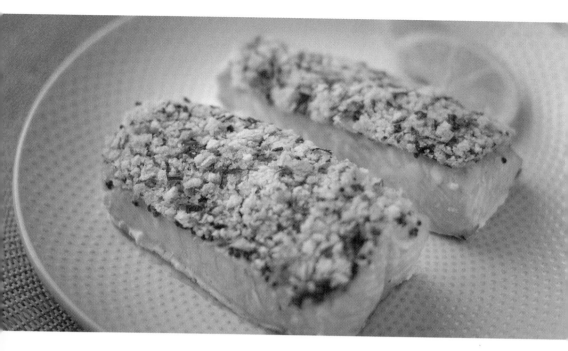

Salmon with Herb Crust
Serves 4

I entered a version of this recipe into a fish cookery competition when I was in first year Home Economics. It came second and I remember being a bit disappointed that it hadn't won. Even so, this is a really tasty dish and one we eat a lot in our house.

Preheat oven to 180°C.

Line an ovenproof dish with parchment.

Mix the breadcrumbs with the herbs, lemon zest, melted butter and then tip onto a flat plate.

Season the salmon, spread with 1 tsp of the mustard and press into the breadcrumbs until the top is coated. Place into an ovenproof dish on the parchment and chill for about ten minutes.

Remove from the fridge, add about 30ml water to the dish (not on top of the salmon, just around it). Bake for about ten minutes

If you like, you could place under a hot grill at this point to toast the crumbs for about five minutes to make the topping nice and crunchy.

60g breadcrumbs

2 tbsp flat-leaf parsley, finely chopped

2 tbsp chives, finely chopped

zest of half a lemon

20g melted butter

salt and pepper to season (if you use them)

4 salmon fillets

4 tsp wholegrain mustard

Calories: 275kcal

| 7.25g carbs | 1g fibre |
| 21.75g protein | 17.5g fat |

Serving Suggestion:
Serve with sumac carrots or baby potatoes with salsa verde

Thai-style Fish Cakes with Spicy Red Pepper Sauce
Serves 4

These are lovely served with one of the bean or broccoli recipes.

Preheat oven to 180°C.

Chop the fish into 4cm pieces approximately and put into food processor.

Pulse till it becomes a coarse mixture.

Add the rest of the ingredients, except the breadcrumbs, and pulse until combined. Don't over-pulse as you don't want mush.

Shape into patties, press lightly into the crumbs and place on parchment-covered baking tray. Cover in cling film and refrigerate for 30 minutes to an hour. Spray a light spray of oil on them and bake for about 12–15 minutes until done.

Throw the lemon into the oven alongside the fish cakes for the last five minutes of cooking.

Serve with the spicy red pepper sauce.

For the Spicy Red Pepper Sauce
Heat the oil in a pan and add all the ingredients and stir to coat.

Cook on medium heat for a few minutes until the mix starts to soften.

Top up with enough water to cover and then cook until the onion and peppers are soft.

Blend and taste. Season if needed.

Cool completely before putting into jars and storing in the fridge.

400g salmon, skinned and boned, or use a mix of any firm-fleshed fish

2 spring onions, finely chopped

1 lemongrass, bottom 2.5cm only, trimmed and chopped finely

2 tbsp fresh coriander, finely chopped

1 tbsp lime juice

1 tsp fish sauce

1 tsp tamari or coconut aminos (or soy sauce)

20g breadcrumbs

Gherkins to serve (optional) and a large wedge of lemon

Spicy Red Pepper Sauce

1 tsp oil

2 precooked red peppers, deseeded and roughly chopped

2 red chillis, deseeded and chopped finely

2 tbsp tomato puree

2 cloves garlic, finely mashed

1 medium white onion, chopped

2 tbsp Worcester sauce

2 tbsp white wine vinegar

150ml water

Calories: 253kcal

9g carbs	1g fibre
21.5g protein	14g fat

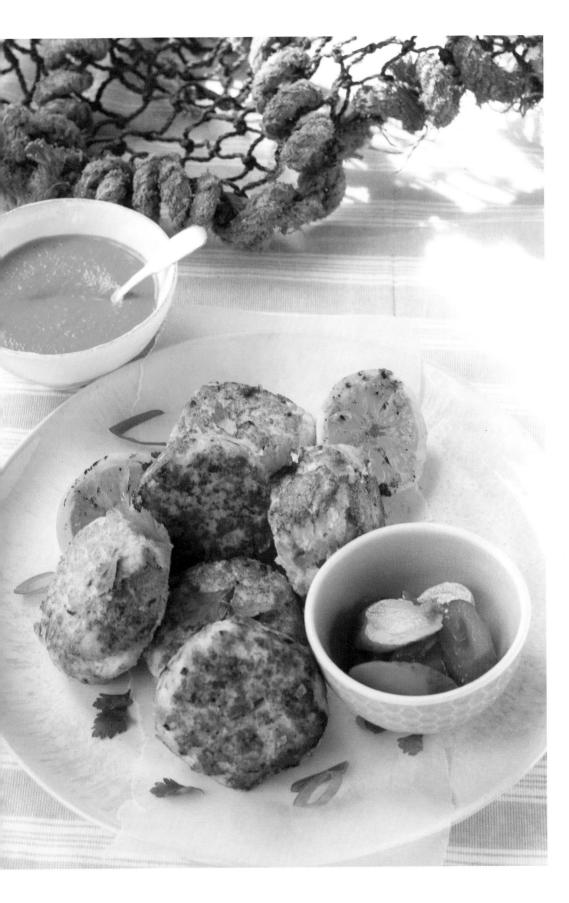

Halibut Provençale and Green Beans
Serves 2

This is the perfect dish when having friends over for dinner: tasty, easy to prepare and looks really appetising on the plate.

Preheat oven to 180°C.

Check the halibut for pin bones, dry with some kitchen roll and season with salt and pepper, if using.

Bring a small pot of water to the boil and blanch the beans for two minutes.

Tip them straight into ice water to seal the colour and stop the cooking. Drain and set aside.

Heat the oil in a hot ovenproof pan and place the halibut into the pan, skin side down.

Keeping the pan quite hot, allow the skin to crisp. Don't move the fish around the pan. After about two minutes move the pan into the oven to finish the cooking (depending on the thickness of the fish it should be done in about eight minutes).

Meanwhile add the tomatoes, chilli flakes and sugar to a pot and cook for two minutes. Blend well to a smooth sauce and keep warm.

Take pan out of the oven and remove the fish to a warm plate. Put the beans into a pan with a little hot water to warm through for a minute or two. Lay out two serving plates and spoon the tomato sauce onto each. Arrange the beans on top, then place fish onto the beans and dot over the tapenade.

2 pieces of halibut

salt and pepper

4 handfuls of green beans, trimmed

1 tbsp rapeseed oil

½ x 400ml tin tomatoes

pinch of chilli flakes

pinch of sugar

2 tbsp good-quality olive tapenade

Calories: 293kcal

6g carbs	2g fibre
16.5g protein	22g fat

Serving Suggestion:
Serve with the butter bean or chickpea mash if you wanted something a little more substantial.

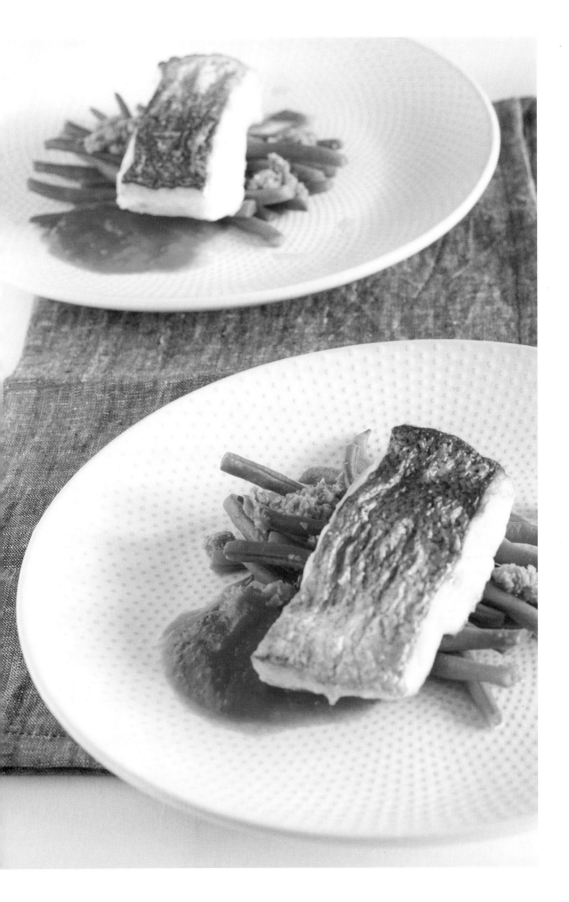

Miso-glazed Sesame Salmon
Serves 4

This is a quick and easy recipe and very popular in our house. I always keep a jar of miso paste handy in the fridge.

Preheat oven to 180°C.

Whisk together the miso paste, mirin, honey, garlic, ginger and mustard.

Place salmon into a dish, spread over the marinade and leave for 30 minutes (or longer in the fridge if you have the time).

Spray a large baking tray with some oil, place the salmon skin side down. Add the asparagus and season everything with salt and pepper, if using. Reserve two spoonsful of marinade and drizzle the rest over the salmon. Sprinkle with the sesame oil and sesame seeds and bake for around ten minutes until the salmon is done to your liking. Halfway through, baste the salmon with the rest of the marinade.

15g miso paste

50ml mirin

1 tbsp honey

2.5cm piece of ginger, peeled and grated

1 clove of garlic, finely mashed

1 tsp wholegrain mustard

4 salmon fillets, skin on, descaled

1–2 sprays oil, for the baking tray

360g small asparagus, trimmed

salt and pepper

1 tsp sesame oil

2 tbsp sesame seeds

Calories: 316kcal

19g carbs   3.5g fibre   24g protein   16g fat

Serving Suggestion:
Serve with sweet potato mash

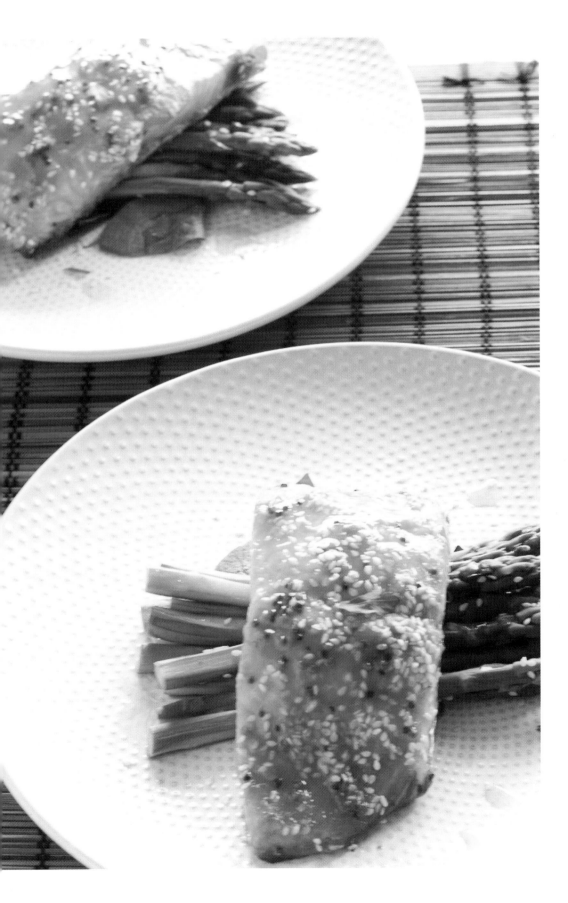

Tuscan Bean Salad with Tuna
Serves 4

Preheat oven to 180°C.

Lightly grease a baking tray with some oil and roast the cherry tomatoes, cut side up, for 15 minutes. Set aside until needed.

Heat the oil over a medium heat. Add the onion, garlic and rosemary, and cook gently until softened (about five minutes). Add the beans and season with salt and pepper, if using. Stir in the balsamic vinegar and cook for about three minutes until everything is warm.

Divide the beans across four plates.

Drain the tuna, add to the beans and divide the cherry tomatoes across the plates.

8oz cherry tomatoes, halved

½ tbsp oil

1 small onion, chopped finely

2 cloves garlic, finely mashed

1 tsp chopped fresh rosemary

1 tin each haricot and cannellini beans (480g total)

salt and pepper, if using

5 tbsp balsamic vinegar

400g tin of tuna (I use tinned in water)

Calories: 230kcal

| 19g carbs | 7g fibre | 39.5g protein | 2.2g fat |

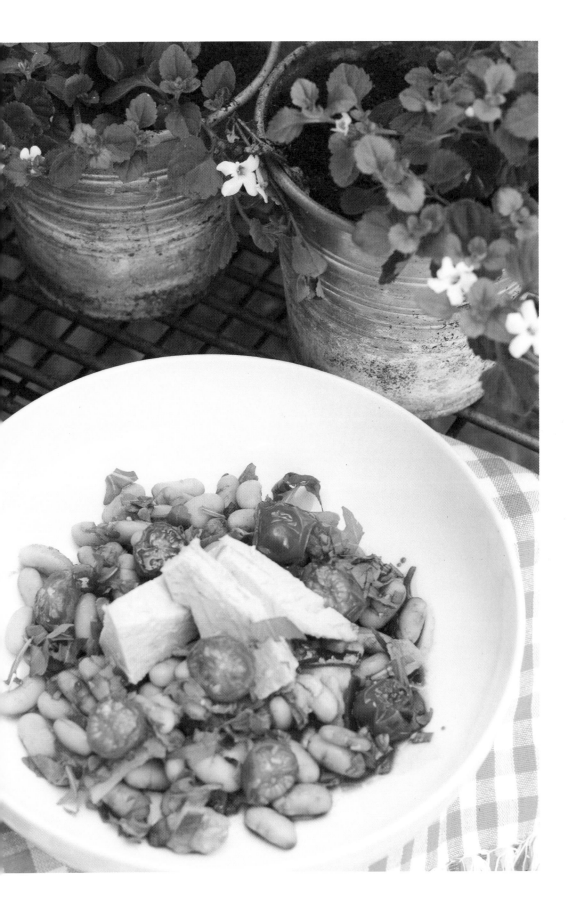

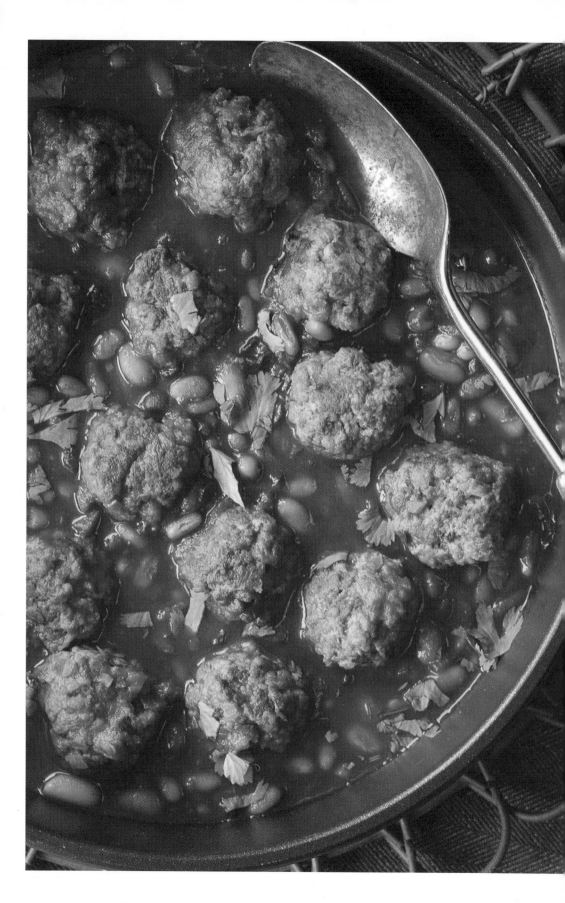

Mexican-style Meatballs with Bean Stew
Serves 6

This Mexican-style recipe is very popular in our house. I have listed the name of my online supplier where I stock up on chillies, chipotles and other Mexican ingredients. An alternative ingredient is given below – it won't quite be the same but will be delicious nonetheless!

Preheat oven to 170°C.

Place the ancho chilli into the warm stock to rehydrate, then remove the seeds and chop up quite finely.

Mix the beef, breadcrumbs, egg and coriander, and form into meatballs (approximately 18).

Add a few sprays of oil to a pan and brown the meatballs on all sides. Move to a dish and set aside.

Add onion to the pan and cook over medium heat until almost soft. Add garlic and cook for another minute. Splash over a bit of stock if it seems dry.

Stir in the puree, paprika, vinegar and sugar and stir to incorporate. (Add the ancho chilli substitute here if not using ancho chilli.) Cook for a minute.

Add the stock, the drained beans, the ancho chilli and passata, and season well. Bring to the boil, then place the meatballs in the sauce, cover the pan with some tinfoil and pop into the oven. Cook for about 30 minutes, removing the foil for the last ten minutes. (Alternatively, continue to cook on the hob over a low–medium heat, turning the meatballs from time to time.)

Stir in a final handful of chopped coriander, squeeze over the juice of half a lime and, if you wish, a spoonful of natural yoghurt with some grated lime zest over the top before serving.

1 dried ancho chilli (this adds a lovely mild, sweet, smoky flavour. If you don't have it you could add 1tsp mild chilli powder or smoked paprika.

250ml beef stock, warmed – a stock pot or stock cube is fine

600g lean beef mince

60g breadcrumbs

1 egg

3 large handfuls fresh coriander, chopped

1 medium white onion, chopped

2 cloves garlic, finely mashed

2 tbsp tomato puree

1 tbsp sweet paprika

1 tbsp white wine vinegar

1 tbsp brown sugar

350ml tomato passata

salt and pepper

1 400g can each of kidney and cannellini beans (or 2 tins of your choice)

handful of fresh coriander, chopped

juice and zest of ½ lime

natural yoghurt

Calories: 263kcal

18.5g carbs	7.5g fibre
27.5g protein	7g fat

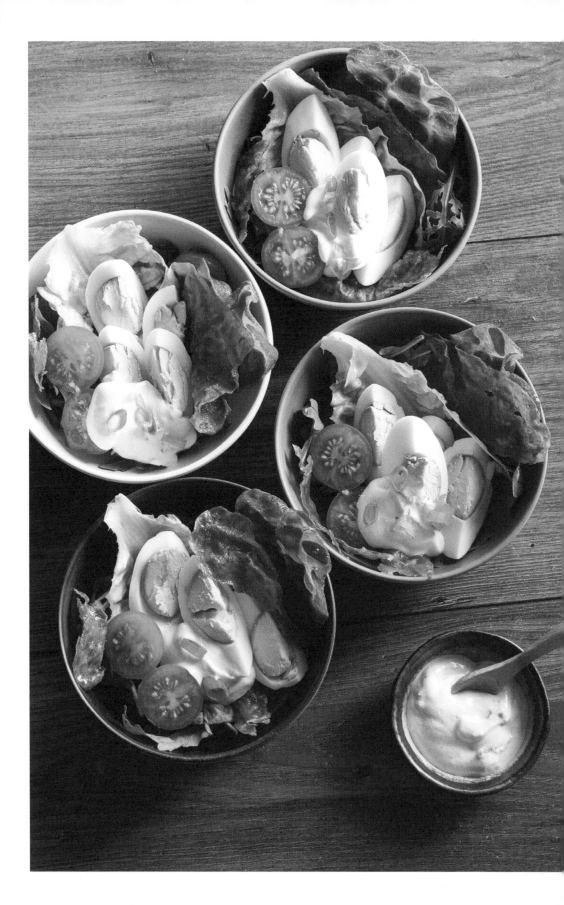

Special BLT Salad with Egg and a Dijon Dressing
Serves 4

I love this simple salad. The dressing has a delicious kick from the anchovies. Grilling the ham makes it lovely and crispy. Top with a grilled chicken breast for an even more substantial evening meal.

Boil the eggs and quarter them.

Grill the ham until crispy (which will be about one minute a side under the grill).

Make the dressing by combining everything and whisking together well.

Separate the baby gem into leaves.

Arrange all the salad leaves onto four plates, add the eggs and tomatoes.

Break the ham into big pieces and scatter over the top of the eggs.

Drizzle the dressing over and serve.

8 eggs

8 slices Parma ham or spicy salami

2 small baby gem lettuce heads, stalk removed and washed

4 handfuls of rocket

8 cherry tomatoes, halved

For the dressing

3 anchovies, finely chopped

2 tbsp white wine vinegar

2 tbsp lemon juice

4 tbsp natural Greek-style yoghurt

2 tsp Dijon mustard

Calories: 207kcal

| 3g carbs | .5g fibre | 19g protein | 13g fat |

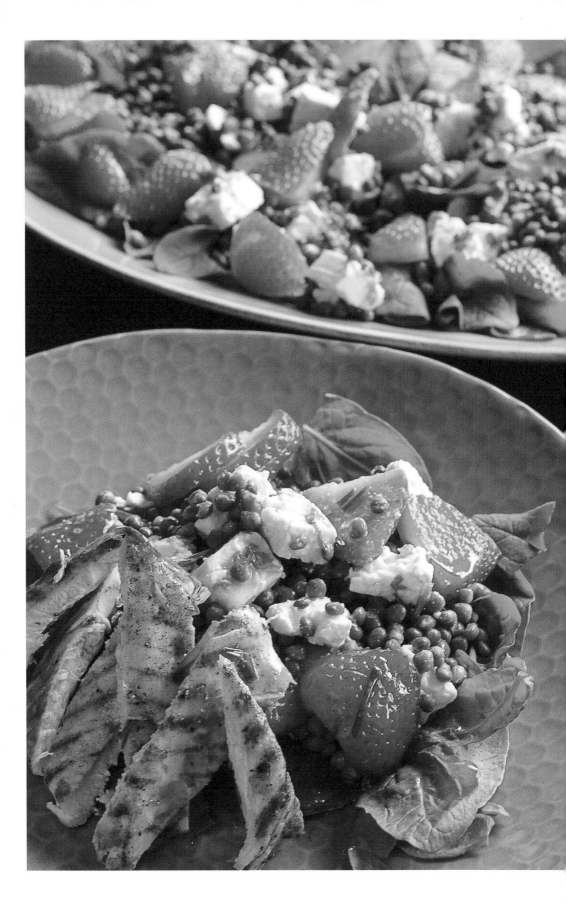

Grilled Chicken Breast with a Spinach, Lentil, Strawberry and Feta Salad
Serves 4

This is a delicious salad and is a complete meal. It works perfectly to take to work or school for lunch also.

Blend all the dressing ingredients, taste and season if necessary, then set aside until the salad is ready.

Rinse the lentils, place in a pot and cover with cold water. Bring to the boil, turn down to simmer and cook for about 20 minutes until tender.

Meanwhile, toss the chicken in the oil and cook on a griddle pan (or frying pan) for about five minutes a side until perfectly done. Slice and set aside and keep warm while you finish the lentils.

Drain the lentils and allow to cool slightly then add the chopped feta, spinach and sliced strawberries. Season and pour over the dressing and gently mix to incorporate.

Divide across four serving plates and top with the cooked chicken breast and serve.

250g green lentils (or you can use any you prefer)

4 chicken breasts, flattened

½ tsp rapeseed oil

100g feta cheese, crumbled or chopped into small slices

100g (small bag) of spinach, cleaned and drained

200g strawberries, washed, hulled and sliced

salt and pepper, if using

For the dressing

juice and zest of ½ lemon

2 tbsp white wine vinegar

25ml extra virgin olive oil

1 tbsp honey

1 handful of mint leaves, chopped finely

Calories: 470kcal

39.5g carbs   10.25g fibre   46g protein   13.5g fat

Spiced Lentils with Spinach
Serves 4

Legumes on their own are not a complete protein so if you are eating this without adding some meat or fish, you should instead add some grains, seeds or nuts to make it complete. Use any split peas or lentils you like. Simply follow the instructions for cooking as per the packet.

Cover the rinsed lentils in water or stock, bring to the boil, then turn down to a simmer and cook until tender. This is usually 20–30 minutes and can be done ahead: they will sit happily in the fridge, covered, for a day or two.

Meanwhile, heat the oil, add the onion, garlic and chilli, and cook gently until softened.

Stir in all the spices and let cook for a minute or two to remove the rawness. If it looks a bit dry, just add a splash of water.

Stir in the tomato puree and cook for a minute, stirring. Add the coconut milk and tomatoes. Stir to combine and bring up the heat to medium. Cook for about five minutes. Taste and season if needed.

Add the lentils, stir in the spinach and cook gently. At this point if it is a little thick, simply add some water or stock.

Sprinkle the chopped coriander on top and add a squeeze of lime juice and serve.

200g red split lentils, soaked and rinsed

2 sprays of cooking oil

1 small onion, chopped finely

2 cloves garlic, finely mashed

1 tsp mashed chillis or 1 small red chilli, deseeded and chopped finely

1 tsp nigella seeds (omit if you can't find)

1 tsp coriander

1 tsp cumin

1 tsp mild (or hotter if your family likes it) curry powder

1 tsp garam masala

½ tsp turmeric

1 tbsp tomato puree

1 400ml tin light coconut milk

½ x 400g tin chopped tomatoes

100g frozen spinach or 1 small bag of fresh spinach

3 tbsp fresh coriander, chopped

juice of ¼ lime

Calories: 278kcal

| 39g carbs | 5g fibre | 15.25g protein | 8g fat |

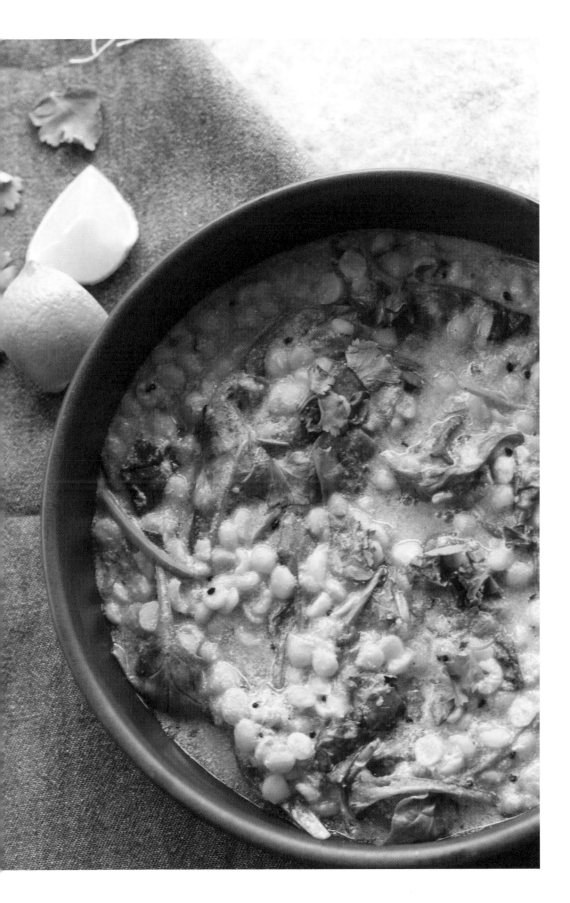

Spicy Chickpea and Butter Bean Burgers
Serves 2

We make a version of bean burgers most weeks.

Preheat oven to 180°C.

Place all the ingredients bar the oil and the breadcrumbs into a food processor, season well and whizz until it forms a rough paste. Don't overdo it.

Divide the mixture into four portions. With a light touch, form into patties and flatten slightly. Dip in the breadcrumbs and chill for 15 minutes.

Heat a pan with two sprays of oil and lightly brown the cakes on both sides.

Transfer to a baking tray lined with parchment and finish in the oven for about ten minutes.

1 x 400g tin butter beans, drained and rinsed

1 x 400g tin chickpeas, drained and rinsed

2 spring onions, finely chopped

1 tbsp fresh mint, chopped

1 tbsp coriander, chopped

zest of a lime

1 tsp harissa paste

1 tbsp coconut aminos, or you can use soy sauce or tamari as an alternative

60g breadcrumbs

2 sprays of cooking oil for the pan

Serving Suggestion: Serve with Asian slaw or roasted cauliflower.

Calories: 192kcal

26g carbs   11g fibre   10g protein   2.5g fat

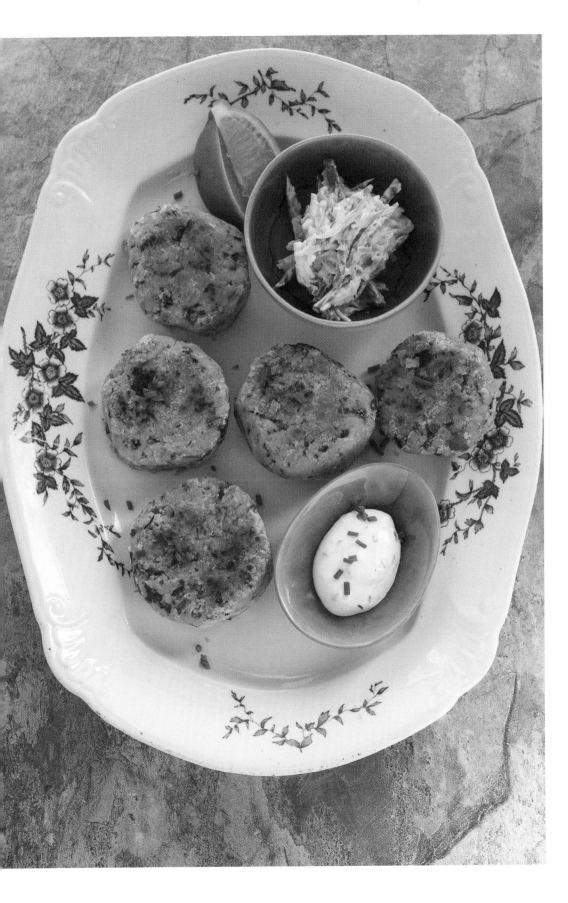

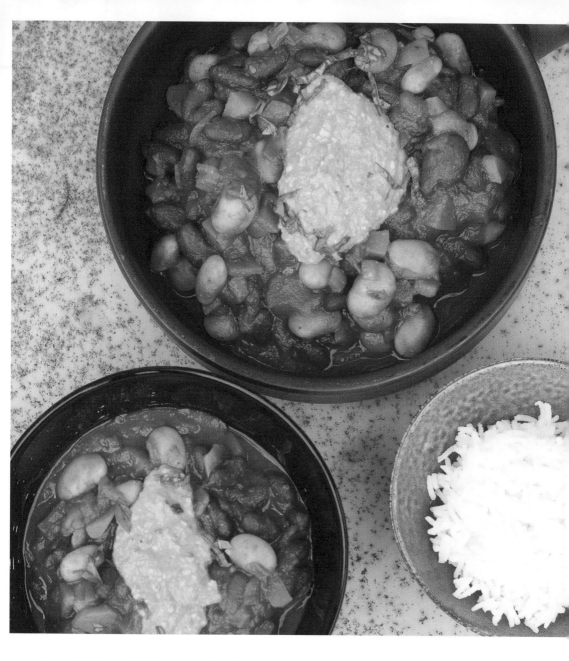

Mixed Bean Bolognese with Tomato Rouille
Serves 6

The secret to a good bolognese is to cook low and slow. Gently simmer for at least 30 minutes and the flavours will be intensified. This bolognese is a great, easy option for midweek. Being plant-based, it is super for your health.

Calories: with rouille and rice 371kcal

50g carbs	9.5g fibre
13g protein	10.5g fat

Heat the oil and toss in the garlic, onion, celery and carrot. Add 10 ml of water, stirring to coat. Turn the heat down to medium and cook for about ten minutes. You want a trace of brown on the edge of the vegetables.

Add the oregano and southern-style spice mix, stir to coat well and cook on a low heat for a few minutes. If it is dry, add a splash of water.

Add the tomato puree. Stir well and then add the drained tomatoes and the tomato passata. Cook for about 15 minutes over a low heat. Add the beans and the Worcester sauce, stir well and cook until the beans are fully heated through and the flavour has developed. If possible leave this for at least another 15 minutes to cook over a low heat.

Serve with a spoon of the tomato rouille dolloped on top and a portion of rice.

Tomato rouille

This keeps in the fridge for a few weeks and is delicious with any meat fish or roasted veg. It is amazing on top of this dish. It is high in calories but you are only using a spoon or two at a time and it is full of good fats.

Place the tomatoes on an ovenproof dish, season and drizzle a tiny bit of olive oil over them.

Place the garlic, still in the foil, alongside the tomatoes and roast for 20 minutes until the tomatoes begin to char.

Squeeze the garlic out (use edge of a knife on each clove if very hot) into the bowl of a food processor, add everything else and blend well.

Taste and adjust the seasoning as you wish.

Cool and decant into a jar and store in the fridge.

½ tbsp oil

2 cloves garlic, finely mashed

1 small onion, finely chopped

1 celery stalk, cleaned, trimmed and finely chopped

2 medium carrots, washed, trimmed and finely chopped

1 tsp dried oregano

1 tsp southern-style spice mix (see page 260)

1 tbsp tomato puree

1 x 400g tin tomatoes, drained

400ml tomato passata

3 x 400g tins (drained weight 240g) beans (choose from kidney, cannellini, haricot and butter beans), drained and rinsed

1 tbsp Worcester sauce

rice, to serve

Makes a large jarful

6 small tomatoes, cut in half

80ml olive oil

1 bulb of garlic, halved horizontally and loosely wrapped in tinfoil

100g cooked red peppers (from jar)

50g sliced almonds

50g breadcrumbs

50ml sherry vinegar

2 tsp chopped chilli in oil or 1 fresh chilli, deseeded and chopped finely

salt and pepper, to taste

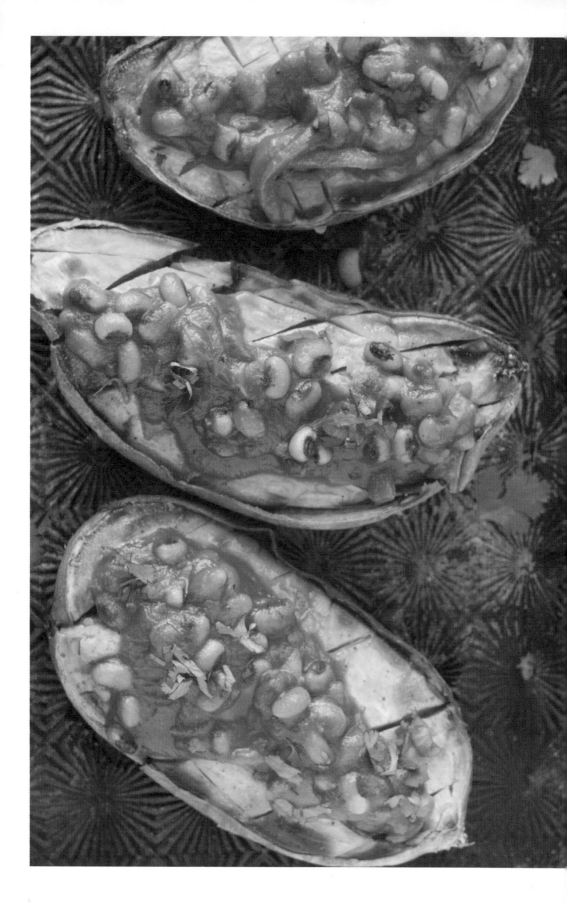

Sweet Potatoes with Spicy Beans
Serves 4

This is a really filling meal, loaded with carbohydrates, so great for replacing lost energy stores after sport, and one the whole family will like.

Preheat the oven to 180°C.

Pierce the sweet potatoes a few times and place in the oven to bake until tender and cooked through (about 30–40 minutes).

Meanwhile, heat oil in a frying pan over a medium heat and add the onion and chorizo and cook until the onion is soft and chorizo has released its lovely oil. This will take about five minutes.

Add the garlic and cook for two minutes, stirring to prevent it from catching. Add a bit of water if it seems dry. Add the spice mix and cook for a minute or two before adding the tomato puree, tomato passata and chipotle in adobo, if you have it. Season well and cook for about two minutes, then add the drained beans.

Reduce the heat to low and cook for about ten minutes to allow the beans to heat and take on the lovely flavours of the sauce. Feel free to add more water if you want to loosen it a bit.

Remove the sweet potatoes from the oven, cut in half and cut across the potatoes a few times to make room for the beans and place on serving plates.

Divide the beans over the sweet potatoes and sprinkle with some chopped fresh coriander and a squeeze of lime juice.

2 large sweet potatoes, washed

½ tbsp oil

1 medium white onion

25g chorizo, in small cubes

1 clove garlic, finely chopped

1 tbsp southern-style spice mix (see page 260) or use 1 tsp of paprika and ½ tsp of cayenne pepper

1 tbsp tomato puree

350ml tomato passata

1 tsp chipotle in adobo – omit if you can't get it. It is delicious but the dish will still be great without it

salt and pepper, if using

1 x 400g tin butter beans (240g drained weight)

1 x 400g tin cannelloni beans (240g drained weight)

1 tbsp fresh coriander, chopped

juice of ½ lime to finish

Calories: 400kcal

72g carbs   17g fibre
15g protein   5g fat

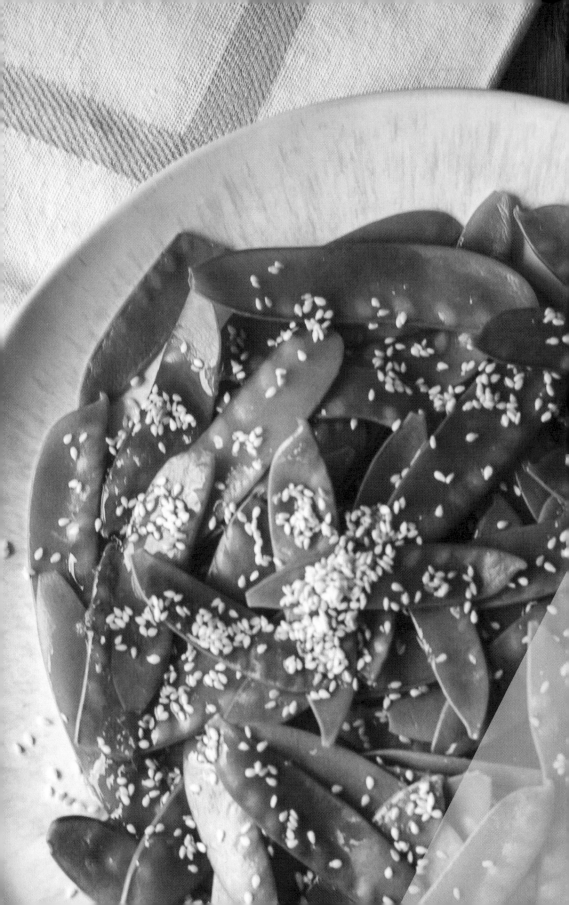

Vegetables/ Side Dishes

I adore almost all vegetables. For me, they are an important part of any meal: the star player, not the side. They should cover the bulk of your plate and since there are so many vegetable options out there you should be able to find some the whole family will love. They are especially great if you are trying to lose weight because they help fill you up – they contain loads of that all-important fibre and because they are relatively low in calories you can eat a good selection of them every day. I use dressings and spices to ramp up the flavour of vegetables and add good fat to my meals.

Finish eating before you feel you've had enough ... your brain needs a minute or two to catch up and realise you are full.

Garlicky Green Beans with Sesame and Nigella Seeds
Serves 4

Blanch the beans in boiling water for three minutes, then drain in cold water – this sets the lovely green colour.

Heat the oil in a pan over a medium heat. Add the nigella and sesame seeds and when they begin to pop, add the garlic, stirring to ensure it doesn't catch. Keep the heat at medium and add the green beans, stirring until they are warm and have taken on the flavour of the garlic and the nigella seeds. Add a splash of water if needed while heating.

You can blanch the veg ahead of time and they will keep in the fridge.

Variation: broccoli is also delicious like this. Substitute the green beans with 1 head of broccoli, cut into florets, which have been blanched or steamed ahead of time to almost cooked.

400g green beans, trimmed

½ tbsp oil

1 tbsp nigella seeds

1 tbsp sesame seeds

2 cloves garlic, finely sliced

Calories: 60kcal

| 9g carbs | 3g fibre | 2.5g protein | 2g fat |

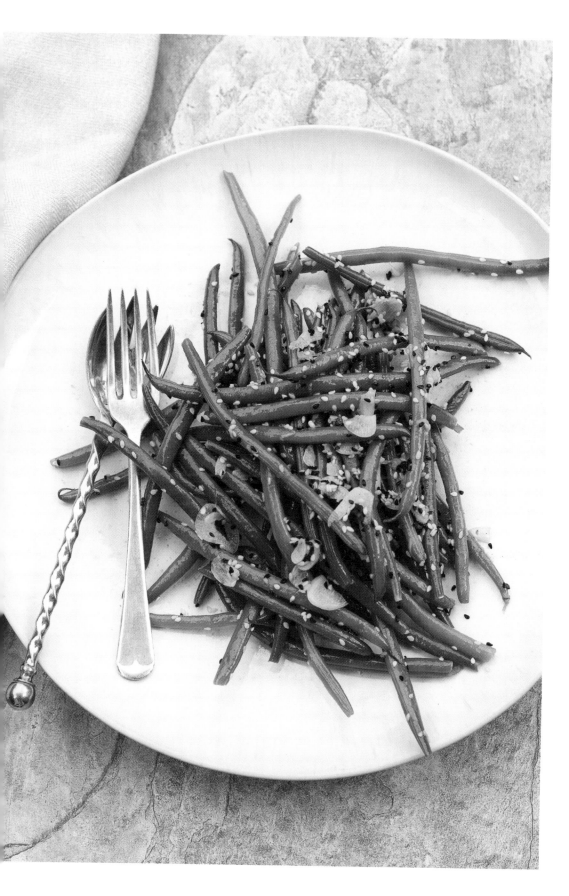

Mangetout or Green Beans with Sesame and Ginger Dressing
Serves 4

The secret to this recipe is to keep a crunch in the veg so don't overcook!

Wash and trim the ends of the beans. Place in a steamer over a saucepan of boiling water. Cover and steam for three to four minutes or until beans are tender but still crunchy.

Place dressing ingredients in a screw-top jar and shake well to combine.

Arrange beans on a plate and drizzle over the dressing. Sprinkle with the seeds and serve.

Variation: you could also make this with 250g steamed or blanched broccoli and it is just as delicious.

250g mangetout or green beans

Dressing

1 tsp finely chopped fresh ginger

3 tsp extra virgin olive oil

1 tsp toasted sesame oil

1 tsp honey

1 tsp tamari or coconut aminos (or soy sauce as an alternative)

2 tbsp toasted sesame seeds

Calories: 135kcal

10g carbs   1.75g fibre   2.25g protein   10g fat

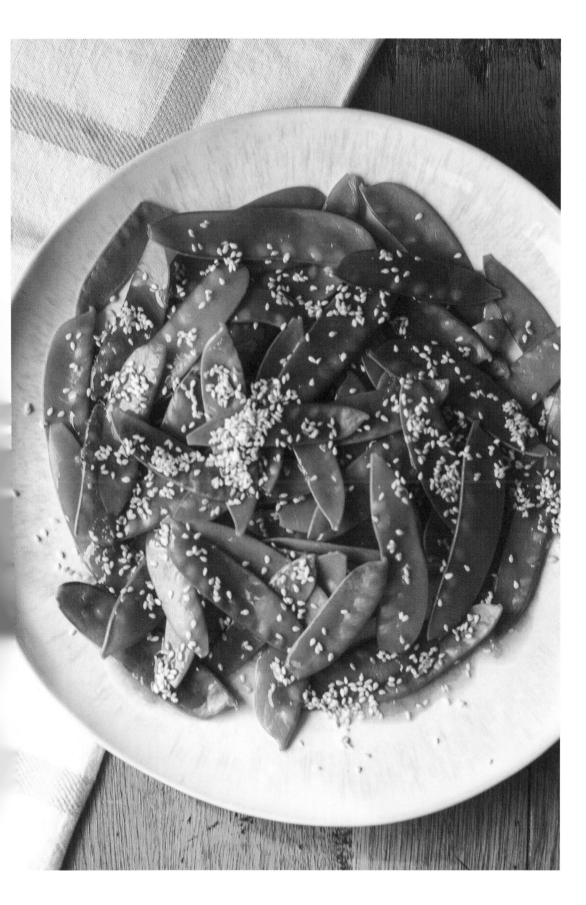

Broccoli with Hazelnut Vinaigrette and Pistachios
Serves 4

The nut oil coats the broccoli, giving it a delicious flavour. You can also use walnut or sesame oil – equally delicious.

Blanch the broccoli or steam until just tender. Drain well.

Whisk the lemon juice with sugar and garlic and season with salt and pepper, to taste. Whisk in the oils and vinegar until well emulsified and add the red onion.

Pour the vinaigrette over the broccoli.

Sprinkle the chopped pistachios and herbs on top.

250g tender-stem broccoli, trimmed and washed

juice of a lemon

pinch of sugar

1 garlic clove, finely chopped

salt and pepper

1 tbsp hazelnut oil

2 tbsp olive oil

½ tbsp balsamic vinegar

½ red onion, finely sliced

10g pistachios, chopped

1 tbsp fresh mint, finely chopped

1 tbsp flat-leaf parsley, finely chopped

Calories: 109kcal

6.5g carbs   2g fibre   2g protein   8.5g fat

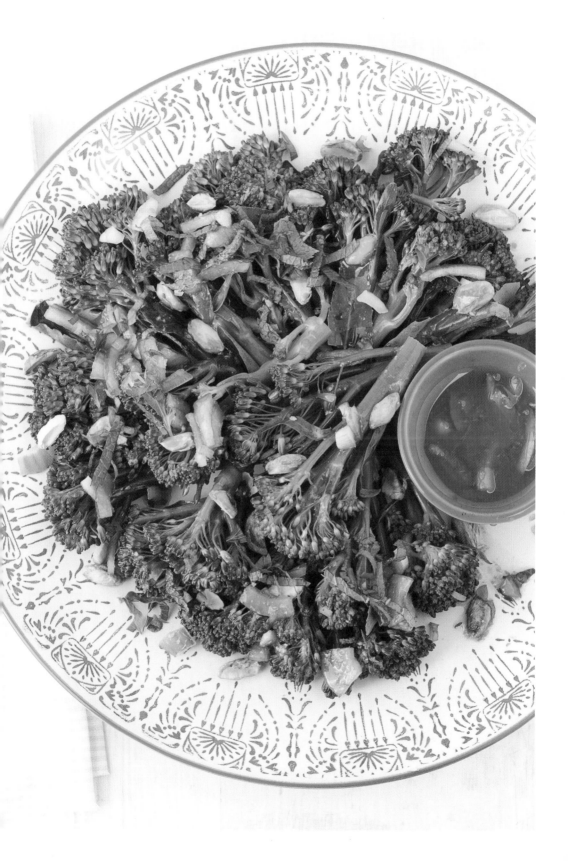

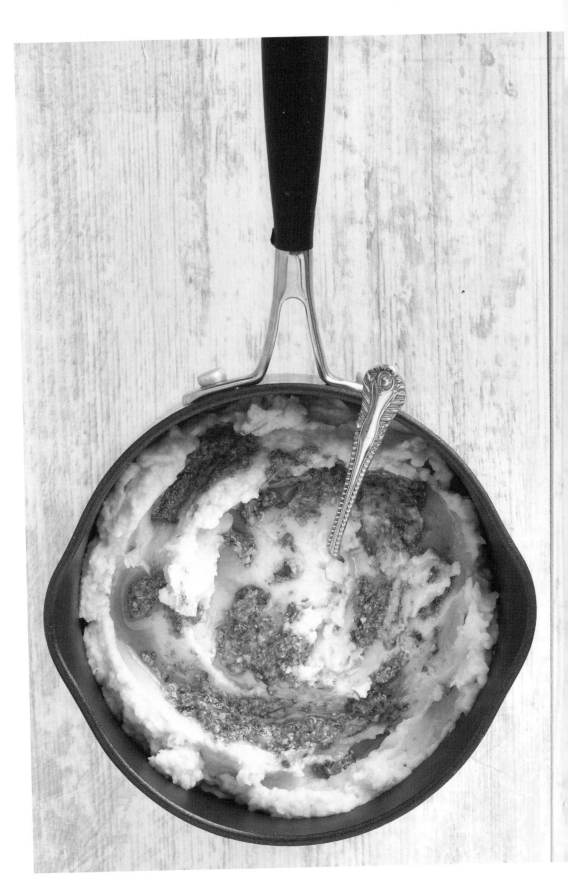

Butter Bean Mash with Basil Oil
Serves 6

Heat the oil and cook the garlic and shallot over a gentle heat until softened.

Drain the butter beans, tip into a blender and add the onion mix. If the consistency needs to be loosened, add in some hot water, or stock if you have it. Taste and season if necessary.

Put into a pot and warm through, then drizzle over the basil oil just before serving.

Calories: 72kcal

8g carbs	4g fibre
4g protein	2g fat

A few sprays of oil

1 garlic clove, finely mashed

1 shallot, chopped finely

2 x 400g tins butter beans (480g drained weight in total)

Basil oil

1 handful fresh basil leaves, chopped

1 tbsp olive oil

Simply mix to combine.

Variation: Chickpea Mash with Thyme
Serves 6

Heat the oil and cook the shallot, garlic and thyme over a gentle heat until softened. Add water if needed. Season well. Add the paprika and stir thoroughly to combine.

Drain the chickpeas. Put into a blender and add the onion mix. Add some water if the consistency needs to be loosened. Tip into a pot and warm through just before serving.

Calories: 60kcal

7.5g carbs	3.5g fibre
3.5g protein	1g fat

A few sprays of oil

1 shallot, finely chopped

1 garlic clove, finely mashed

1 tsp chopped fresh thyme

½ tsp paprika

2 x 400g tins chickpeas (480g drained weight in total)

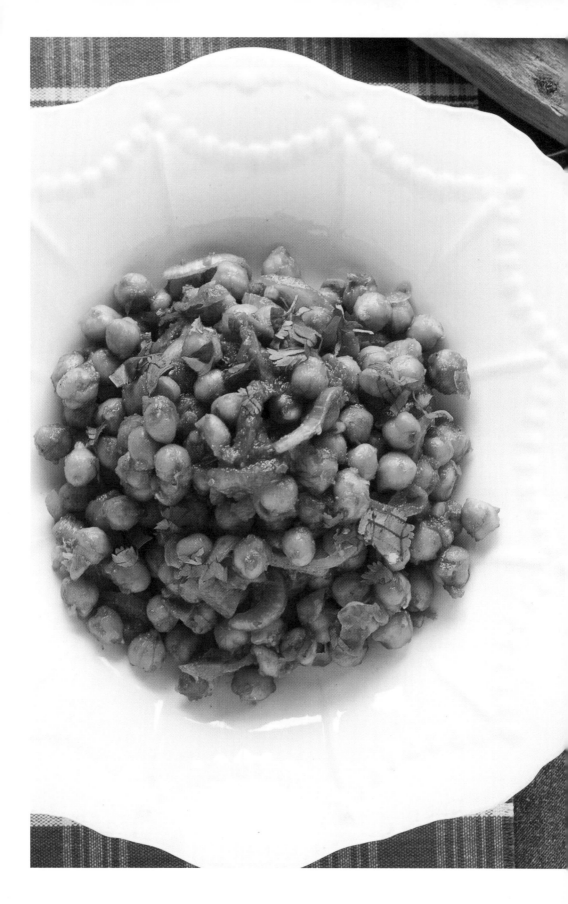

Spiced Chickpeas
Serves 4

Heat the oil, add the onion and cook over a gentle heat until soft and translucent. Add a splash of water if needed. Add the spices and cook for one minute, stirring.

Add the tomato puree and mix well to incorporate.

Add the chickpeas, mix well and season. Cook over a medium heat until the chickpeas are warm and the flavours are developed.

Just before serving, add the chopped coriander and the squeeze of lemon juice.

A few sprays of oil

1 onion, finely sliced

½ tsp cumin

½ tsp coriander

½ tsp garam masala

1 tbsp tomato puree

1 x 400g tin chickpeas, drained

salt and pepper

1 tbsp chopped fresh coriander

a squeeze of lemon juice

Calories: 57kcal

8.25g carbs   3g fibre   3g protein   .75g fat

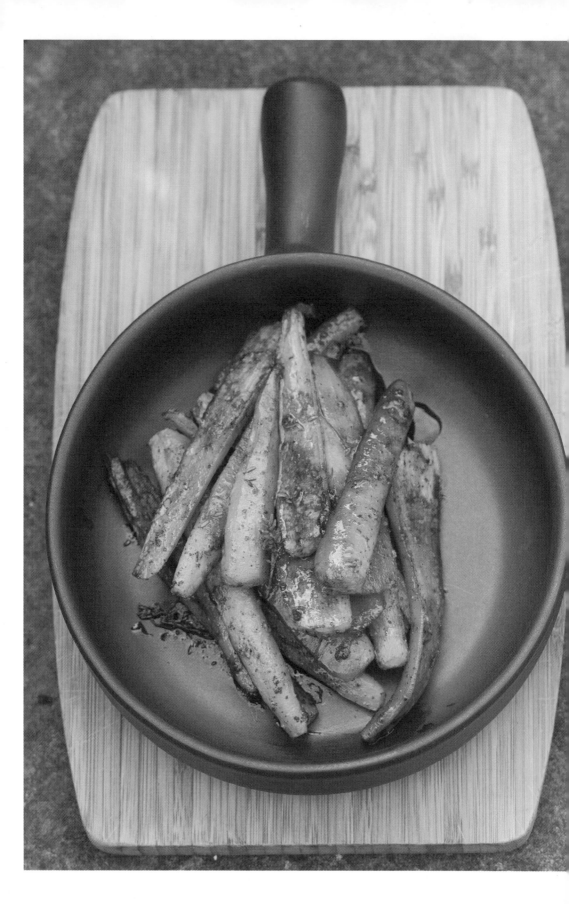

Sumac Roasted Carrots
Serves 4

Preheat oven to 180°C.

Place carrots, thyme, garlic, oil, sugar and sumac into a bowl and toss to coat. Season with salt and pepper.

Tip onto a tray and roast for about 20 minutes until tender. Remove from the oven, squeeze out the garlic onto the carrots (use the tip of a knife for doing this if, unlike me, you don't have asbestos fingers!) and mix to combine.

Mix the sherry vinegar and molasses. Drizzle the carrots with the dressing and toss to coat, then serve.

300g carrots, washed and trimmed into batons

1 tbsp chopped fresh thyme

3 garlic cloves, skin on

2 tbsp olive oil

1 tbsp coconut palm or dark brown sugar

1 tsp sumac (this is a berry which is dried and has a wonderful tangy lemon flavour. If you can't get it, substitute with 1 tsp lemon zest.

salt and pepper

1tbsp sherry vinegar

1 tbsp pomegranate molasses

Calories: 104kcal

15g carbs   2.5g fibre
.75g protein   5g fat

Variation: Carrots with Ras-el-Hanout
Serves 4

Preheat oven to 180°C.

Place carrots, oil, ras el hanout and salt in a bowl and toss to coat.

Tip onto a tray and roast for about 15 minutes. Drizzle over the honey and cook for a further ten minutes until tender.

300g carrots, washed and trimmed into batons

2 tbsp olive oil

1 tsp ras-el-hanout

½ tsp salt

1 tbsp honey

Calories: 99kcal

13g carbs   2.25g fibre
.75g protein   5g fat

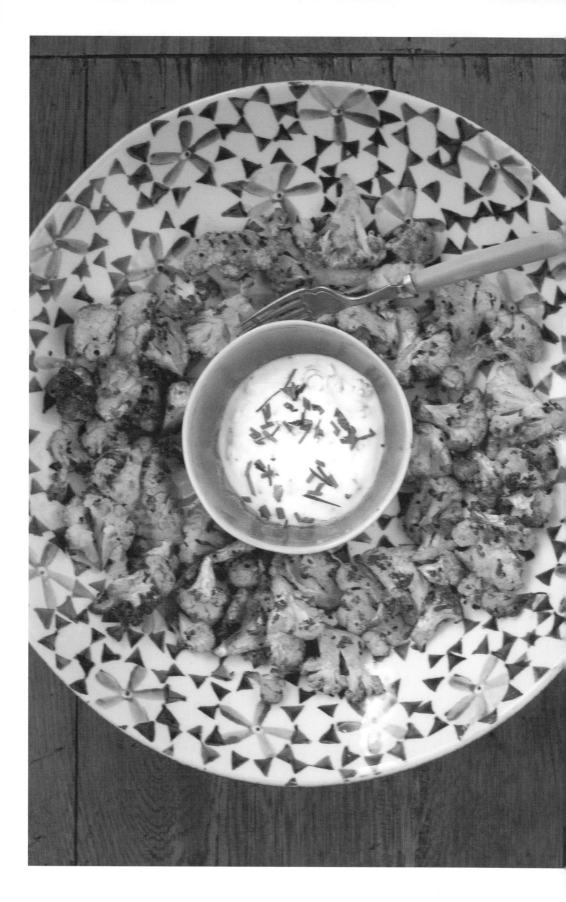

Roasted Cauliflower with Yoghurt Dip
Serves 4

Cauliflower is my favourite vegetable, hands down. This recipe is for four but I probably could eat the whole thing in one sitting!

Preheat oven to 200°C.

Mix the spices and oil and stir well to combine.

Toss in the cauliflower and mix well to coat with the spice mix.

Spread out on a baking tray and roast for about 20 minutes.

For the Yoghurt Dip

Mix yoghurt with garlic. Stir in the herbs.

Add lemon juice and season if needed.

Serve with the roasted cauliflower.

Calories: 100kcal

8g carbs	3g fibre
2.5g protein	6.5g fat

1 tsp cumin

1 tsp salt

1 tsp curry powder

1 tsp nigella seeds

½ tsp turmeric

2 tbsp oil

400g cauliflower, in bite-size florets and slices

Yoghurt Dip

3 tbsp Greek-style natural yoghurt

1 clove of garlic, finely mashed

1 tbsp coriander, chopped

1 tbsp chives, chopped

1 tbsp mint, chopped

1 tbsp lemon juice

Spiced Greens
Serves 4

I use kale in this recipe but it will work equally well with any other greens you like, such as cabbage or spinach. If you use spinach, don't precook.

Blanch kale in boiling water for two minutes, remove and drain well, then chop.

Heat the oil in a medium-sized pot. Add the onion and a drop of water, and cook, lid on, until soft.

Stir in the spices and cook for about a minute. Add a splash of water if needed, then add the puree and tin of tomatoes, as well as a tin of water. Add the kale, pressing down as needed until it reduces in the sauce. Season well and cook for about ten minutes over a low–medium heat until some of the tomato sauce has thickened and the flavours are developed.

150g kale, cleaned and any big stalks removed

2 sprays cooking oil

1 small white onion, diced

1 tsp turmeric

1 tsp nigella seeds

½ tsp cayenne

½ tsp ground cumin

½ tsp ground coriander

1 tbsp tomato puree

1 x 400ml tin tomatoes

salt and pepper

Calories: 59kcal

11g carbs   1g fibre   2.5g protein   .5g fat

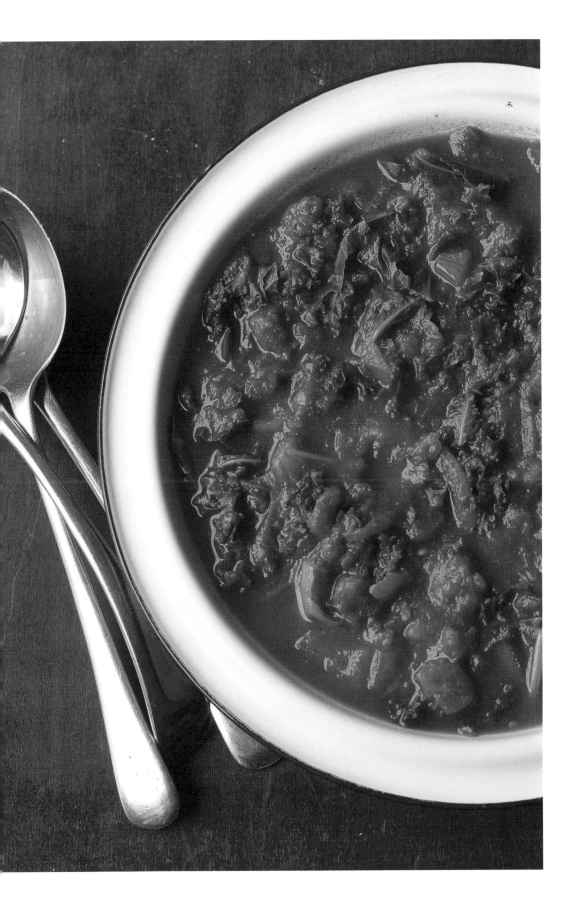

Baby Potatoes with Salsa Verde
Serves 4

These potatoes are just amazing with some salsa verde spooned over.

Cover the potatoes with cold water, bring to the boil, then simmer until tender.

Drain and, using a potato masher or large spoon, gently crack the potatoes slightly – don't smash them completely.

Tip into a bowl and, while warm, stir in the salsa verde. Mix well and serve.

400g baby potatoes, washed

3 heaped tbsp salsa verde (see page 256)

Calories: 155kcal

18.5g carbs   1g fibre   2g protein   8.5g fat

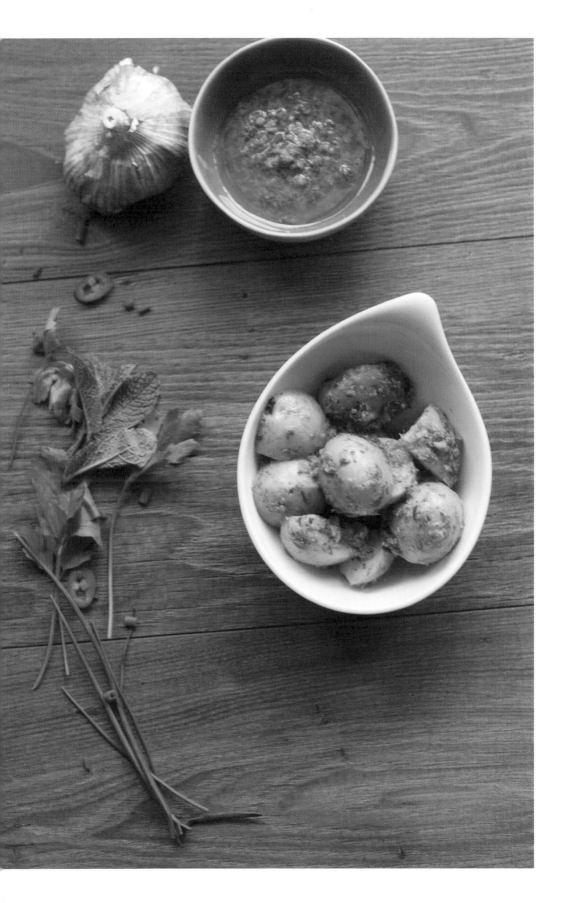

Spicy Sweet Potato Mash
Serves 4

Peel and cut the sweet potatoes into equal size pieces. Add to a pot of water, ensuring the water covers them. Bring to the boil and simmer until tender.

Drain, and reserve a cup of the water.

Tip the sweet potato into a blender, add the harissa and coriander and season well.

Blend, adding some of the cooking water if needed.

Taste and, if you need to up the heat further, add some more harissa paste.

Variation: this can be made with many other root vegetables, such as parsnip, squash, turnip, and would be just as gorgeous. A sage leaf would be amazing with parsnip or turnip instead of the coriander.

4 medium or 2 large sweet potatoes (approx. 800g)

2 tbsp harissa paste

2 large handfuls fresh coriander

salt and pepper

Calories: 185kcal

40g carbs   6g fibre   4g protein   .5g fat

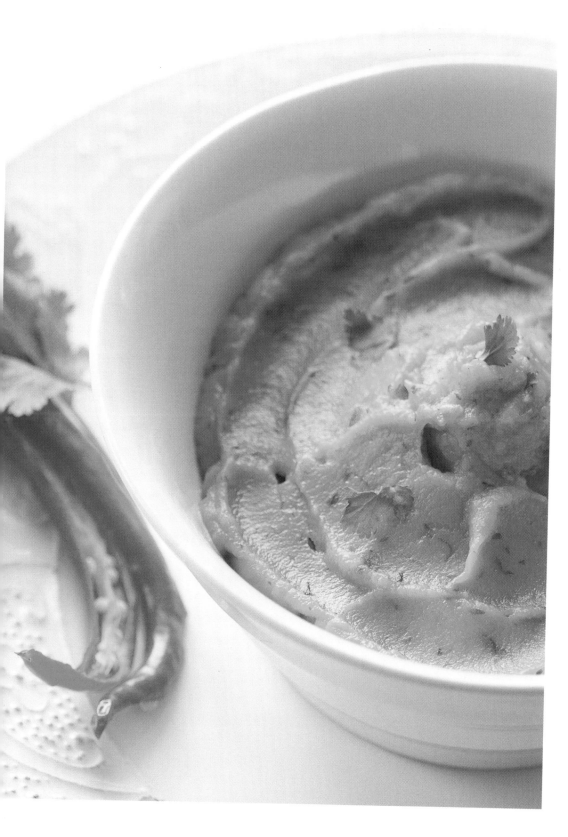

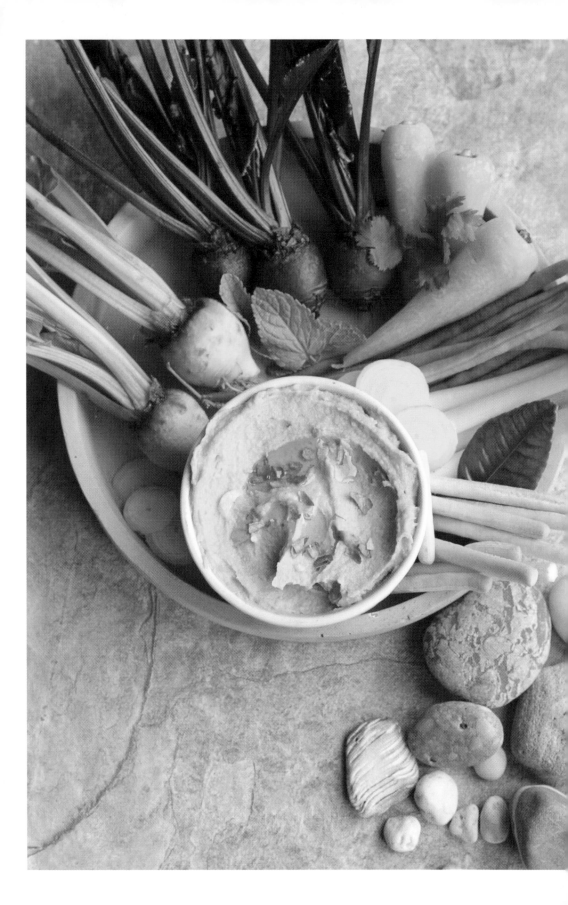

Spicy Sweet Potato Ghanoush
Serves 4

Like an aubergine dip but with sweet potato and, in my opinion, even more delicious. This is great for lunch with boiled eggs and some cooked chicken or fish. I like to cook extra sweet potato and make this with the leftovers. It's also amazing as a dip with some crunchy veg.

Tip everything into a blender and blend until smooth.

Taste and season if needed.

400g cooked sweet potato

60g tahini

1 cooked red pepper from jar

1 heaped tsp mashed red chillis or
½ red chilli, deseeded and chopped

1 tsp sesame oil

½ tsp celery salt

Calories: 200kcal

| 22g carbs | 4g fibre | 5g protein | 10g fat |

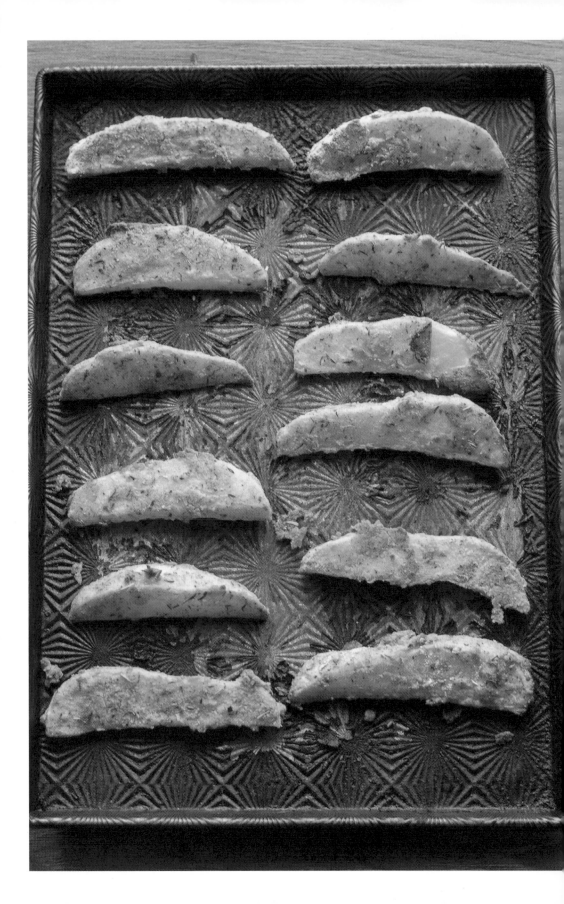

Mojo Potato Wedges
Serves 6–8

I have been making these for as long as I can remember although I no longer remember why I call them Mojo potatoes. I remember making these with loads of dips at a housewarming party years ago and in the early hours of the morning making more of them because they were so popular. This flour mix makes enough to cover six big potatoes or two very large sweet potatoes for between six to eight people. Double as necessary if you need to make more but don't overcrowd the trays or they will steam and not crisp off.

Preheat oven to 220°C – nice and hot.

Mix flour with all the herbs and seasonings and lay out on a large plate

Tip the milk and egg into a wide bowl and mix to combine.

Add the potatoes to the milk, then onto the plate of seasonings, turning until well coated.

Lay the potato wedges on parchment on a baking tray (or straight on the tray with a light spray of oil). Bake for ten minutes, then flip over and bake for ten more.

100g flour

½ tsp dried thyme

½ tsp dried basil

½ tsp dried oregano

½ tsp black pepper

½ tsp chilli powder

½ tsp garlic salt

1½ tsp paprika

½ tsp cayenne

100ml milk

1 egg, beaten

6 big white potatoes or 2 large sweet potatoes, cut in wedges

Calories: 222kcal

47.5g carbs	5g fibre	6g protein	1g fat

Note: the calorie profile is only slightly higher with sweet potato and has more fibre.

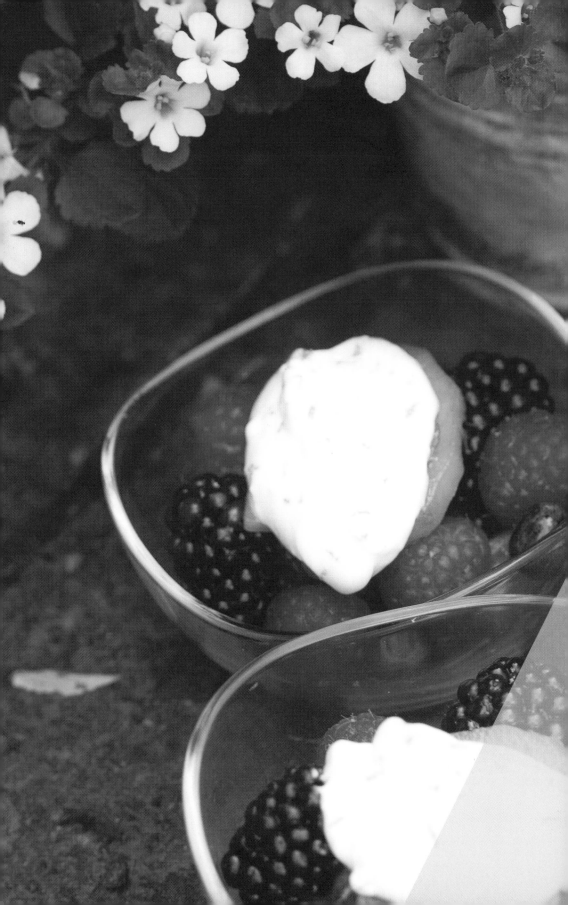

Desserts and Sweet Things

Desserts are not something we have every day in our house, and while I hate the word 'treat' to describe them, we usually only have dessert at the weekend if we are having people over.

Neither of us believes that too much sugar should feature in anyone's diet, regardless of how active you are. There is also a lot of talk about how one sugar is better than the other. Our take on it is that sugar is sugar, you should know your intake and not eat too many things containing sugar regardless of how so-called healthy you are told it is.

If you want to have dessert or cake occasionally, then do. If possible, make it yourself and that way you'll know what goes into it, there won't be any strange additives or preservatives to improve shelf life and, if it's served with love, then the joy to be had from an occasional dessert is worth it. Guilt shouldn't come as a side order with food, so know what you are eating, enjoy it and don't eat the lot.

Don't be the person who knows the calories in everything but the taste of nothing.

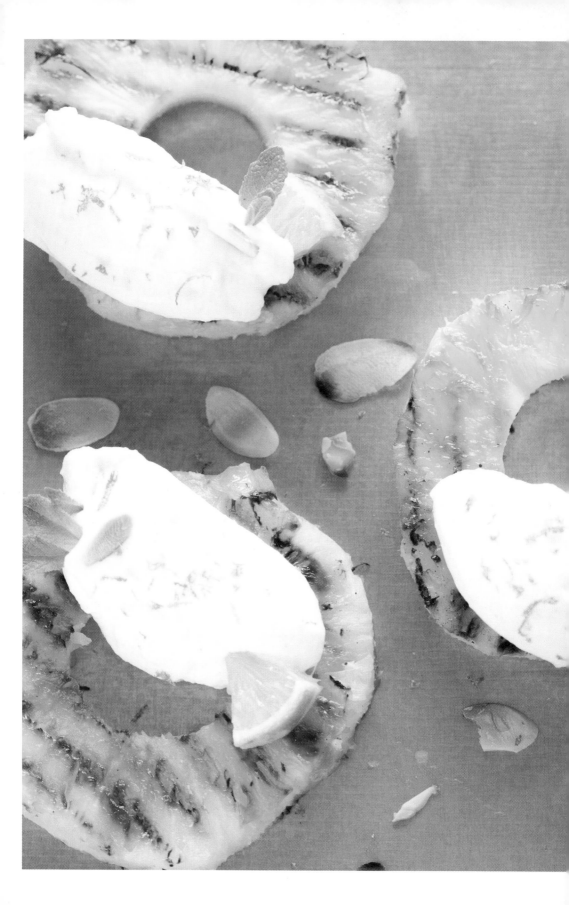

Roast Pineapple with Ricotta Cream
Serves 6

This is a simple, delicious dessert and relatively low in calories, as far as desserts go. If it is summer you could also prepare the pineapple on the barbeque if you have one going. Preparing the pineapple this way means the fruit sugars caramelise into a lovely golden on the pineapple and it is perfect with the ricotta cream topping.

1 pineapple, skin removed, centre stalk removed and cut into 6 rings

250g ricotta cheese

25g icing sugar

juice of 1 lime and the zest of half

Calories: 133kcal

| 17g carbs | 1g fibre |
| 4.5g protein | 5g fat |

Prick the pineapple rings with a fork to encourage some of the juices to run.

Heat a griddle pan and place pineapple rings on it and cook over a medium–hot heat until they start to brown and caramelise. Flip over and do the same the other side.

Meanwhile beat the ricotta with the sugar and add the lime juice and zest.

Serve a pineapple ring with a tablespoon of ricotta cream on top and add an extra sprinkle of lime zest.

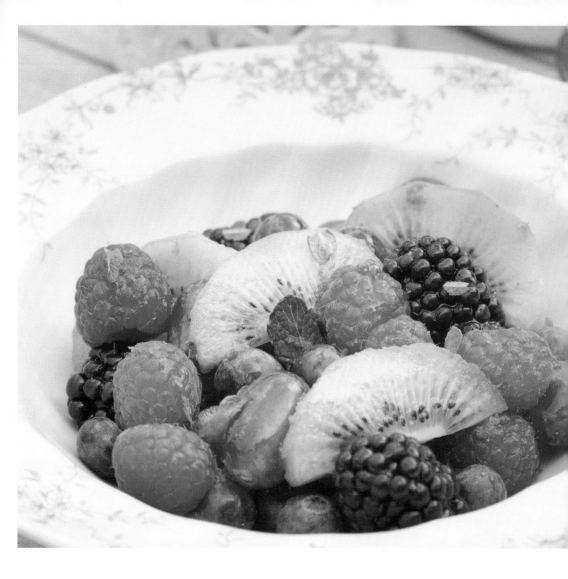

Fresh Fruit Salad Two Ways
Serves 4

The simplest of desserts but there is nothing more glorious than a plate of fresh in-season fruit. You can interchange the fruit as you like. I love blackberries as they are great for fibre – pretty much all fruit is but they are higher. Calories are much the same across raspberries, blueberries, grapes and kiwi, with strawberries and blackberries coming in a bit lower per 100g.

For the apple and lime dressing

Mix the honey and apple juice together.

Add the lime zest and then the juice. Stir well to incorporate.

Prepare the berries and fruit by cleaning as needed and add to a serving bowl.

Pour the apple and lime dressing over and serve.

For the creamy cheesecake topping

Beat the cream cheese, icing sugar, lime juice and zest together.

Spoon the fruit into four serving bowls, and top each with a quarter of the cheesecake topping and an extra sprinkle of lime zest.

With an apple and lime dressing

1 tbsp honey

40ml apple juice

zest and juice of 1 lime

400g mixed berries of choice (raspberries, blueberries, blackberries, grapes and kiwi)

Calories: 75kcal

17g carbs   4g fibre
1g protein

With a creamy cheesecake topping

180g low-fat cream cheese

25g icing sugar

juice of 1 lime and zest of half

400g mixed fruit of choice (raspberries, blueberries, blackberries, grapes and kiwi)

Total calories: 145kcal

21g carbs   4g fibre
5g protein   5.5g fat

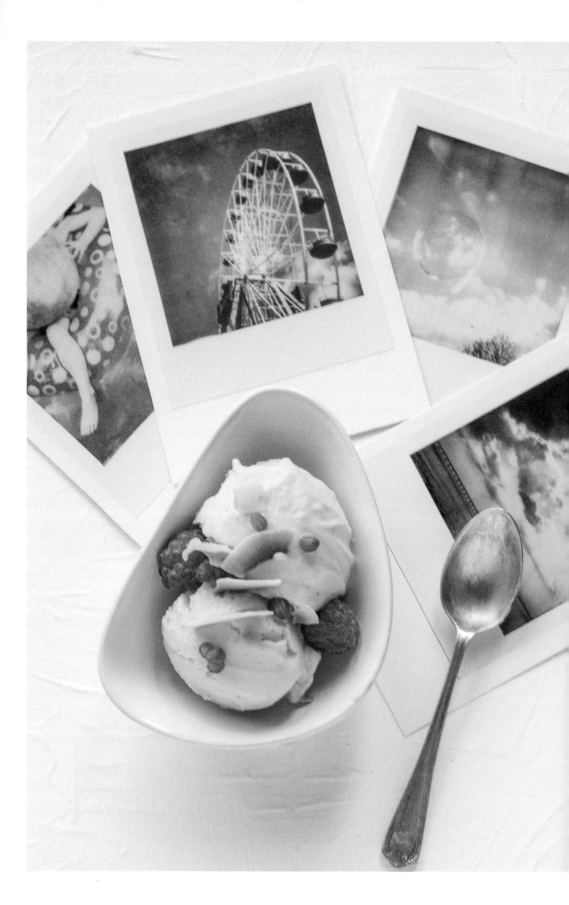

Easy Ice Cream
Serves 6

This simple ice cream is easy to make and the calorie hit is so much kinder when you just use frozen fruit and some yoghurt. I keep bags of frozen fruit handy in the freezer for this. You don't have to stick to the fruit I suggest: experiment with your favourites. Since there are no additives and stabilisers like shop-bought ice cream, it won't keep as long, so make it and use it within a few days!

Place the bananas and mangos onto a flat tray and open-freeze until the fruit is frozen.

Tip into a blender with the yoghurt and blitz until the fruit is completely smooth. You will need to scrape the blender down a few times while doing this. It can be served at this point, or cover the top with a piece of parchment and store in the freezer until needed.

Serve with a handful of raspberries and some toasted coconut.

Mango, Banana and Toasted Coconut Soft-serve

4 bananas, chopped into 2cm-thick slices

2 mangos, peeled and chopped into 2cm-thick slices

100g pot of Greek-style natural yoghurt

125g raspberries

15g coconut shards, toasted

Calories: 129kcal

27g carbs   3g fibre

2.5g protein   1g fat

Mixed Ice Pops

Kids love these ice pops and they are easy to throw together. Ice pop moulds are available in most good kitchen shops. The recipes below make two each.

For the Blueberry
Blend everything and freeze.

Calories: 85kcal

22g carbs   2g fibre

Blueberry

150g Greek-style 0 per cent fat
Blueberry yoghurt

125g blueberries

For the Raspberry
Blend everything and freeze.

Calories: 68kcal

15g carbs   5g fibre

Rasberry

125g raspberries

125g water

1 tbsp honey

For the Raspberry and Pomegranate
Blend everything and freeze.

Calories: 100kcal

24g carbs   5g fibre

Raspberry and Pomegranate

125g raspberries

125g pomegranate juice

1 tbsp honey

For the Coconut Caramel Chocolate
These are more indulgent and will probably appeal more to adults than children.

Add the dates to a pot and just cover with water. Bring to the boil, turn down to a gentle simmer. Cook until very soft. Add the coconut milk, whizz to a paste and let cool, then pour into two ice-pop moulds and freeze. Unmould and cover in 100g melted dark chocolate.

Coconut Caramel Chocolate

100g dates

100ml light coconut milk

100g dark chocolate

Calories: 300kcal

38g carbs   4g fibre
3g protein   13.5g fat

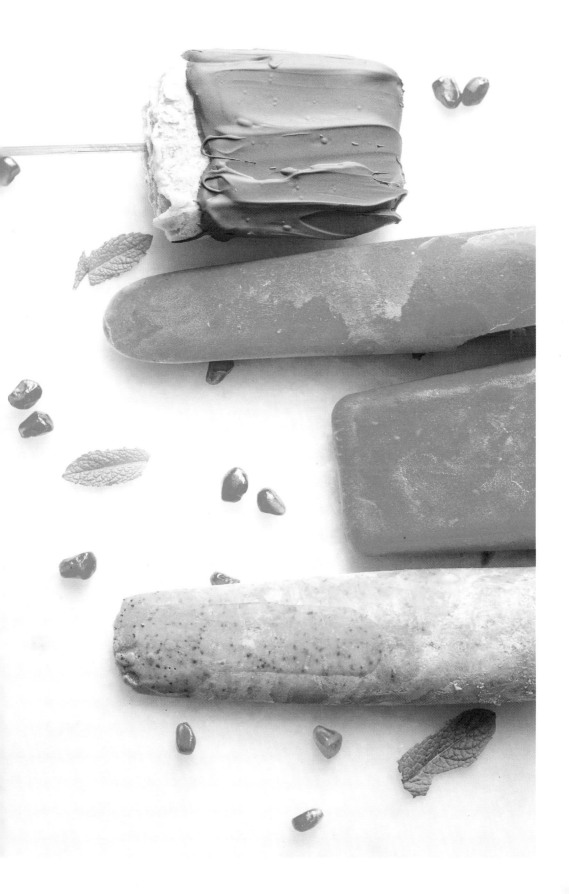

Shortcake Rounds with Fresh Berries
Serves 6

This is a lovely, refined dessert, which I particularly like if I am having people over for dinner.

Preheat oven to 160°C.

Mix flour and cornflour together.

Add the butter and sugar and rub between your fingertips until the mixture is just beginning to come together. Knead lightly until the mixture forms a smooth dough.

Press flat, wrap in cling film and place in the freezer for about 30 minutes.

Tip into blender and blend to breadcrumbs, then pour onto a baking tray and press flat. Cover with some cling film and use a rolling pin to flatten really well, then bake in the oven for about 12 minutes until a very pale golden colour. Mark into six circles with a cutter, then return to the oven for a further six minutes until golden brown. Leave to cool for a few minutes before carefully lifting off onto a wire rack to finish cooling.

Put the fruit into a pot, add the honey or sugar, vanilla and orange juice and bring to a gentle simmer. Cool and then spoon into 6 bowls and top with a shortcake biscuit.

50g plain flour

25g cornflour

50g unsalted butter

25g caster sugar

600g fresh berries or frozen mixed berries

1 tbsp honey or icing sugar

seeds from 1 vanilla pod

juice of half an orange

Calories: 171kcal

28g carbs	5g fibre
2.5g protein	7g fat

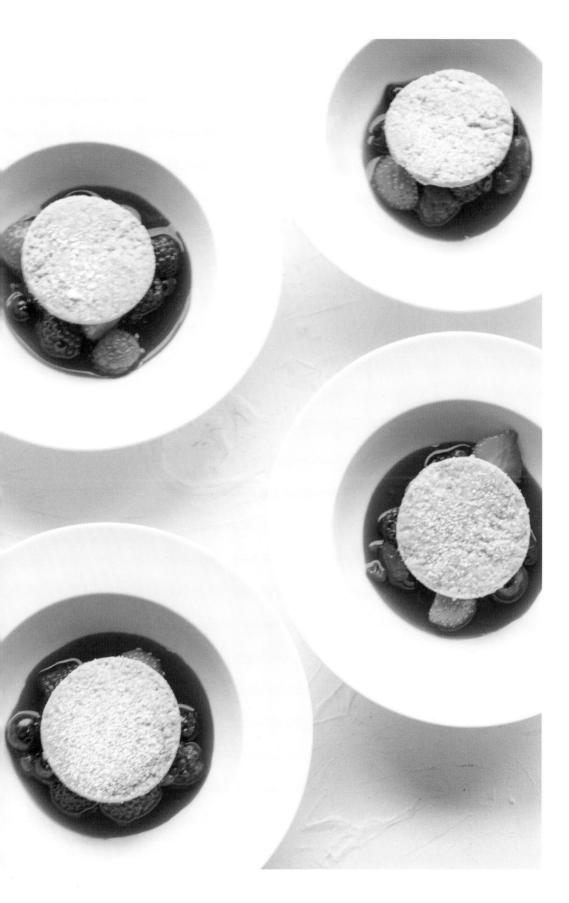

Chocolate and Coconut Cream Pots
Serves 6

This is a decadent dessert – the portion is small but delicious and is plenty. Be sure to use full-fat coconut milk or it just won't set.

Melt the chocolate gently in a bain-marie.

Leave to cool slightly then whisk in the coconut milk until it is fully incorporated.

Pour into small serving glasses – little shot glasses are good.

Top with a sprinkle of hazelnuts and a raspberry, and pop into the fridge for about 20 minutes until set.

110g dark chocolate

170ml full-fat coconut milk

10g toasted hazelnuts chopped

6 raspberries

Calories: 150kcal

6g carbs   2g protein

13g fat

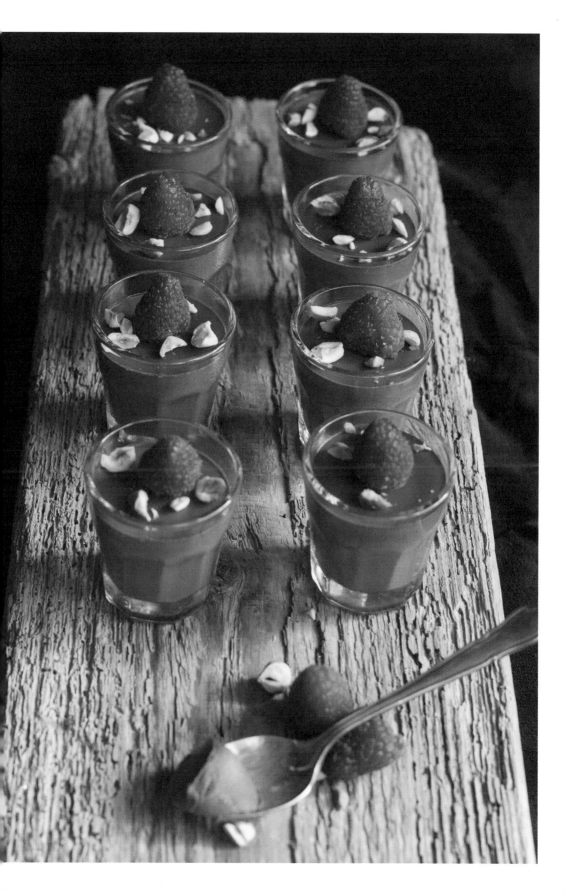

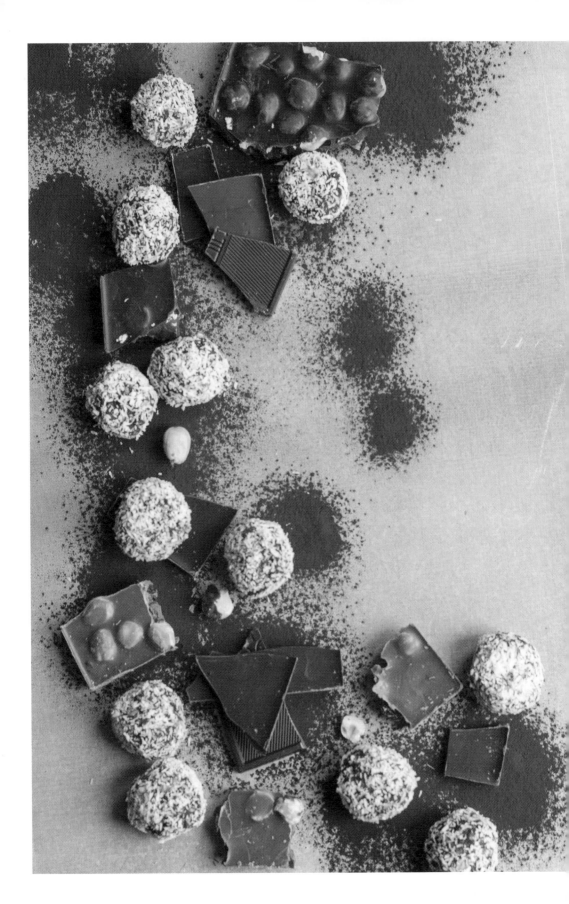

Caramel Crunch Treats
Makes 40

These aren't made on nuts so the calorie hit is much kinder. They are a great option if you want a little sweet on the side with an afternoon tea or coffee.

Preheat the oven to 180°C.

Melt the chocolate gently in a bain-marie.

Chop the dates, put them into a pot and just cover with water. Bring to the boil. Turn down low and gently simmer until they are soft and gooey.

Meanwhile toast the oats in the oven on a flat baking tray until they are golden brown, about ten minutes.

Using a stick blender, blend the dates to a thick toffee paste.

Stir in the oats, followed by the melted chocolate and stir to combine everything well.

Leave it to cool slightly, then roll into small balls, approximately 15g each, and toss them in the coconut.

This will make approximately 40.

Store them on parchment in an airtight container in the fridge.

150g dark chocolate

250g dates

200g oats

25g desiccated coconut

Calories: 61kcal

8.5g carbs

1g fibre

1.5g protein

2g fat

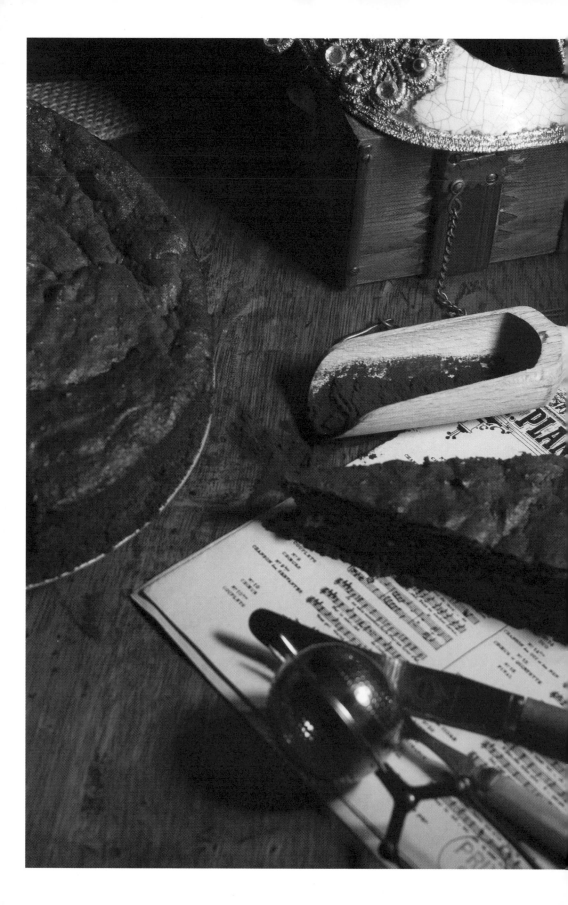

Dark Chocolate and Prune Cake
Makes 14 slices

This is a delicious, rich, decadent cake, perfect for a special occasion. An added bonus is that it is gluten-free. I use only the best of ingredients for this so a small slice is all that is needed.

Preheat oven to 180°C.

Grease and line the base of a 25cm spring-form tin.

Put prunes and water into a pot and simmer gently until the prunes are soft. Blend until you get a thick paste and set aside to cool.

Melt the chocolate with the espresso powder and butter over a gentle heat and stir to combine, stir in the liqueur, if using, then set aside to cool slightly.

Beat the egg yolks, sugar and vanilla together until thick and creamy.

Fold in the prune mixture, followed by the melted chocolate mixture, then the ground almonds.

Beat the egg whites until soft and fluffy and fold into the cake mixture, being careful not to overbeat and take all the air out.

Pour into the tin and bake for 35–40 minutes until a skewer comes out clean.

Cool for about ten minutes, then remove side of the tin and cool fully.

200g prunes, chopped

100ml water

150g good-quality dark chocolate

1 tbsp espresso powder

120g butter

30ml raspberry liqueur (optional)

4 eggs, separated

100g coconut palm or light brown sugar

1 tsp vanilla extract

150g ground almonds

Calories: 265kcal

18g carbs   5.5g protein

19g fat

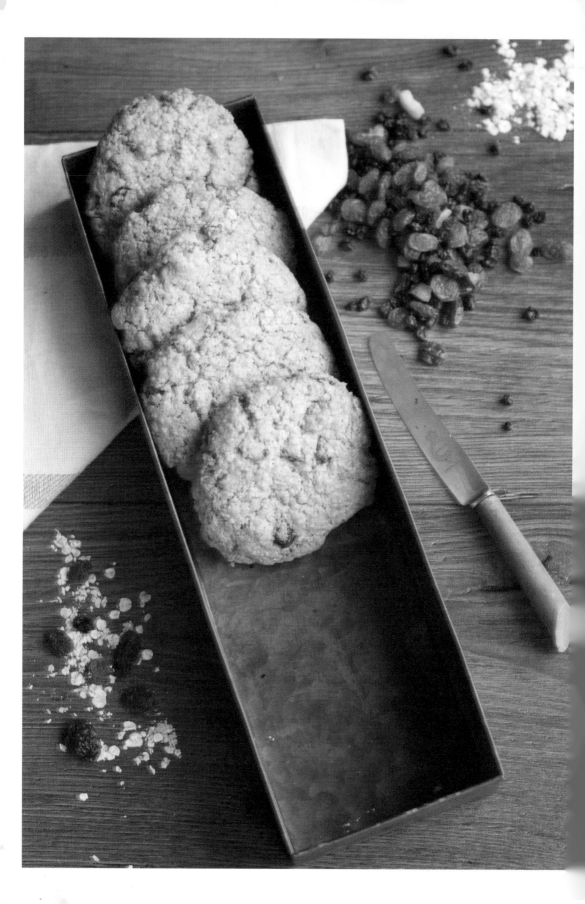

Oat and Fruit Cookies
Makes about 15

Kids love to bake and this is a quick and easy recipe if they want to get the baking bowl out. The ingredients are pretty good and reasonably low on added sugar – still, just have the one!

Preheat oven to 170°C.

Beat the butter and sugar together until soft and creamy.

Add the beaten egg and vanilla, and then stir in all other ingredients and mix well.

Drop rounded tablespoons of the mixture onto a lined baking sheet and flatten slightly.

Bake for 12–14 minutes and allow to cool on the tray. Store in an airtight container.

50g butter, at room temp

75g coconut palm sugar or brown sugar

1 egg, beaten

1 tsp vanilla extract

100g oats

75g chopped figs or other mixed dried fruit of choice

½ tsp baking powder

½ tsp mixed spice

Pinch of salt

Calories: 77kcal

| 10g carbs | 1g fibre | 1.5g protein | 3.5g fat |

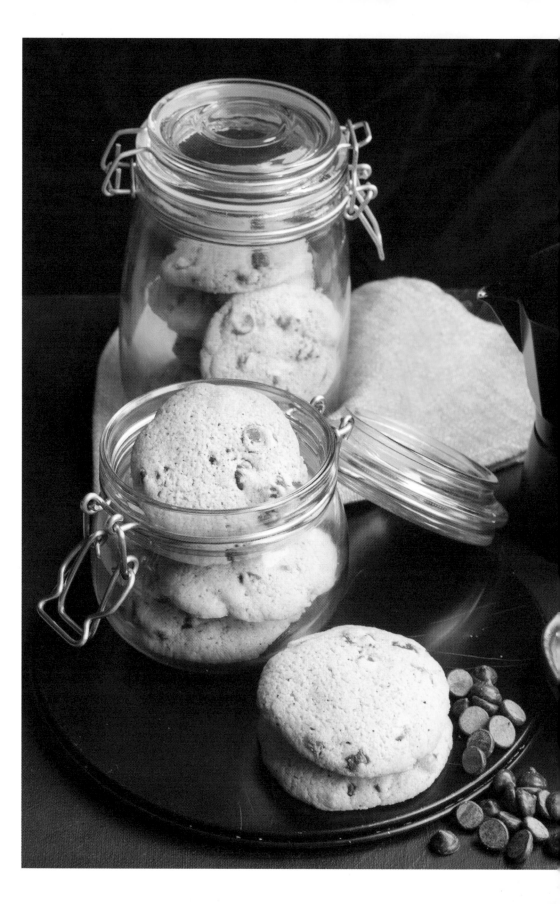

Chocolate chip cookies with sea salt
Makes 20

The espresso powder and pinch of sea salt really enhance the taste of chocolate. These cookies are chewy, chocolatey and a little bit of heaven.

Preheat oven to 170°C.

Mix flour, espresso powder, baking powder and salt together in a bowl.

Beat the butter and brown sugar together until light and fluffy.

Add the egg and beat well.

Gently beat the flour mix into the mixture until just incorporated, then fold in the chocolate chips.

Place tablespoons of the mixture onto baking tray lined with parchment.

Leave space as they will spread. With damp hands, press each down a little, then sprinkle a tiny pinch of sea salt on top.

Bake for about 12 minutes, turning the tray around halfway through.

Remove from the oven and leave for a couple of minutes to crisp up before moving onto a wire rack to cool.

150g plain flour

1 tsp ground espresso powder

½ tsp baking powder

½ tsp salt

100g butter

90g coconut palm sugar or light brown sugar

1 large egg

140g good-quality chocolate chips

sea salt flakes for the top of the cookies

Calories: 120kcal

12.5g carbs   2g protein

7g fat

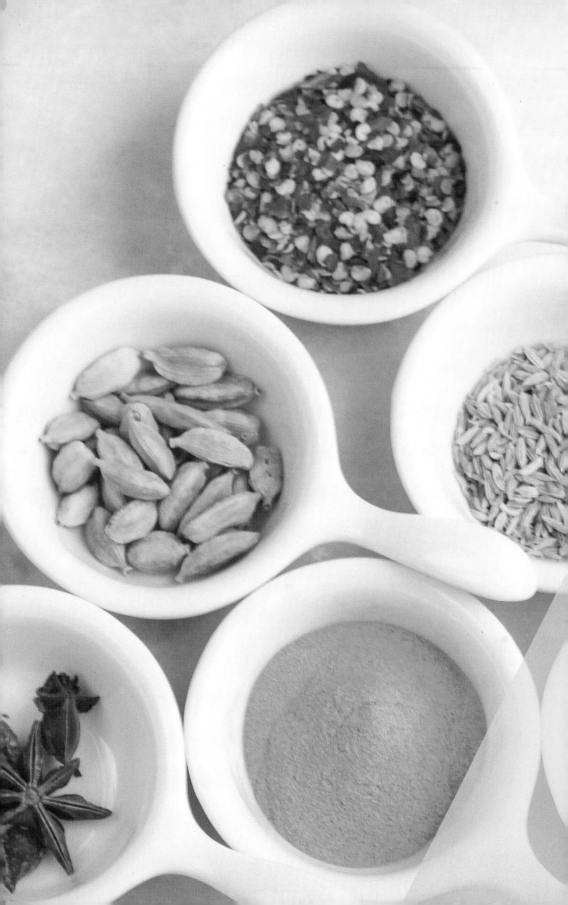

Spices, Sauces, Dressings, Marinades and Dips

I'm all about spices, sauces, marinades and dressings! While there are significant amounts of calories in oils, use them in small quantities. It's worth it for the extra bit of zing they add. I am always willing to forgo dessert if I want to have a lovely dressing or marinade with my food.

Salsa Verde

I have been making this for years. It is a variation on a recipe from the Italian cookery bible *Il Cucchiaio D'Argento*, which I used to be able to read in Italian (I'm rather rusty now, sadly). It is wonderful as a dressing, over chicken or other meat, and is delicious poured over warm veg. I remember making it for a party one time and very late in the night finding some friends dipping crusty bread into the empty bowl to mop up the very last of the juices. This is full of good fat but high in calories so watch the portion size.

Keep aside half the olive oil and put everything else into a food processor.

Whizz for a minute or two, stopping to scrape down from time to time. With machine running slowly, add the rest of the oil.

Taste for seasoning and add salt and pepper as needed.

This will store in an airtight jar in the fridge for a few days.

140ml extra virgin olive oil

2 cloves garlic, peeled and chopped

1 x 50g tin of anchovy fillets

4 tbsp flat-leaf parsley, chopped

2 tbsp each chopped chives, basil and mint

1 tbsp capers

1 tbsp gherkins

1 tbsp lemon juice

salt and pepper, to taste

Peanut Satay Sauce

This is great as a dip or as a sauce on chicken or with turkey kebabs. It can also be stirred into coconut milk and reduced a little for a delicious coconut satay sauce.

Heat the oil in a pan and gently sweat the onion and garlic until soft. Add the rest of the ingredients and stir well to combine. Cook for about three minutes, then blend until nice and smooth. If you prefer it a bit spicy, add 1 chopped and deseeded chilli to the mix when sweating the onion.

½ tbsp oil

½ small white onion, finely chopped

1 clove garlic, finely chopped

200ml water

1½ tsp crunchy peanut butter

1 tbsp sweet soy sauce or 1 tbsp dark soy sauce

1 tbsp brown sugar

juice of ½ lime

Zingy burger sauce

This makes loads and will keep in the fridge. All you need is a spoonful to complete your burger.

Blend everything and tip into a container that can be sealed. Store in the fridge when not in use.

100g crème fraiche

50g mayonnaise

50g tomato ketchup

2 tbsp fresh mint, chopped

2 tbsp chives, chopped

1 tbsp red wine or balsamic vinegar

2 tbsp cornichons, chopped finely

1 tsp paprika

Sweet Chilli Sauce

Delicious with any red meat or chicken.

Heat sesame oil gently, in small pot, add chilli, ginger and garlic, and cook until softened. Add the soy sauce, fish sauce, water and brown sugar. Bring to the boil and simmer for a few minutes. Add the lime juice, stirring well to combine.

Allow to cool then decant into an airtight container and store in the fridge for up to two weeks.

2 tbsp sesame oil

½ chopped red chilli

2 tbsp fresh ginger, finely chopped

1 garlic clove, peeled, chopped and mashed

2 tbsp soy sauce

2 tbsp fish sauce

100ml water

2 tbsp brown sugar

juice of 2 limes

Dukkah

Dukkah is a mix of nuts and spices and there are loads of variations of it. When you are making it, don't pulverise it completely as it should stay quite coarse. Use this to add a crunch to salads, to coat roasted veg or top fish before cooking.

Toast the pistachios until fragrant. Remove to a plate.

Add all other ingredients bar the salt to the pan and toast until fragrant.

Tip out on to the plate and allow to cool.

Coarsely grind with the salt. I use a pestle and mortar but if you have small grinder for spices, it will work. Store in an airtight jar for a week or two.

150g shelled pistachios

4 tbsp sesame seeds

2 tbsp coriander seeds

2 tbps cumin seeds

1 tsp whole black peppercorns

½ tsp salt

Avocado Green Goddess Dressing

Blend everything in a food processor. This will keep for about four days in the fridge.

3 handfuls each of basil, mint and flat-leaf parsley, roughly chopped

3 spring onions, peeled and roughly chopped

1 avocado

2 cloves of garlic, finely mashed

2–3 anchovies from a tin

juice of 1 lemon

1 tsp salt

1 tsp pepper